DIAGNOSIS DEMENTIA

Your Guide for Eldercare
Planning and Crisis Management

NICOLE J. SMITH

DIAGNOSIS: DEMENTIA—III

Diagnosis: Dementia—*Be Aware, Prepare, and Build a Plan of Care; Your Guide for Eldercare Planning and Crisis Management.* Copyright © 2023 by Nicole J. Smith.

ISBN Paperback: 979-8-9890434-0-8
ISBN E-book: 979-8-9890434-1-5

For more information contact
Nicole Smith
PO Box 69864
Tucson, AZ 85755

All rights reserved. No part of this publication may be reproduced, distributed, or transmitted in any form or by any means, including photocopying, recording, or other electronic or mechanical methods, without the prior written permission of the publisher, except in the case of brief quotations embodied in critical reviews and certain other noncommercial uses permitted by copyright law. For permission requests, write to the publisher, addressed "Attention: Permissions Coordinator," at the address above.

The information in this book is not intended as a substitute for consultation with legal, medical, financial, psychological, or governmental experts. Each individual's concerns should be evaluated by a qualified specialized professional.

Cover art: Kristen Graham Brown
Design: Magic Dog Press
Production: Magic Dog Press
Printed in the United States of America

Publisher's Cataloging-in-Publication Data

Smith, Nicole J.

Diagnosis Dementia—Be Aware, Prepare, and Build a Plan of Care: Your Guide for Eldercare Planning and Crisis Management

        p. cm.   photos/illustrations

ISBN: 979-8-9890434-0-8

1. Dementia—Diagnosis 2. Eldercare—Planning— 3. Plan of Care—Documentation 4. Resources—Eldercare Culture

      RC 521 E 93 202   362 196831 Sm

Printed in the United States of America

AUTHOR'S NOTE

In writing this memoir, I drew inspiration from real-life events, yet, in order to respect the privacy of certain individuals, incidents, locations, and entities, I have chosen to fictionalize elements. Any resemblance that may emerge between the names of individuals or events in my book and real-life counterparts is purely coincidental. These details are not meant to portray any actual individual or entity, but rather represent my personal interpretation of the events that shaped my family's story. It's important to acknowledge that others may hold different memories and interpretations of our family's journey.

For my mom

"Whatever you're going through in life, you tend to gravitate towards people who are going through the same things. You can't fix it, but you don't have to go through it alone."[1]

—**Amy Grant,** singer/songwriter
who lost both parents to dementia

---

1 www.agingcare.com/articles/amy-grant-strengthens-faith-confronts-fear-as-family-caregiver-166678.htm

CONTENTS

Author's Note v
Introduction: The Silver Tsunami xv

I. BE AWARE 1

The Dementia Umbrella 1

Signs and Signals 3
   Our Story: The Beginning 4

Behavioral Changes 9
   Evaluation Tools 10
      Our Story: Getting Tested 12
      Our Story: COVID-19 13
   Cooking 16
      Our Story: Food 16
   Driving 17
      Our Story: Driving Miss Crazy 17
   Medication Management 25
      Our Story: Managing Meds 27
   Finances 32
      Our Story: Legal Documents 34
      Our Story: Finances 36

II. PREPARE. 39

Have the Conversation 39
Conversation Starters 41

Legal Documents. 43
Financial Power of Attorney 43
Medical Power of Attorney 45
Guardianship or Conservatorship. 46
Last Wills and Testaments 46
Trusts: Irrevocable, Revocable, QTip .47
Elder Law Attorneys 48

Financial Documents. 49
Beneficiary Designations. 49
Bank Account Cosigners Versus Co-Owners 50
Wealth Advisors 50
Certified Public Accountants. 50
How to Pay for It All 51
Resources for Financial Solutions 53
Books. 53

Critical Contacts Folder. 55
Our Story: Social Security 57

Medical Matters. 63
Do Not Resuscitate. 64
POLST 64

Medications 65
Our Story: Medications 66

Family Dynamics 69
Our Story: Legal Musical Chairs 70
Our Story: Same Play, Different Actors 70

III. BUILD A PLAN OF CARE 75

Don't Go It Alone 75
   Our Story: Hits Close to Home 76

Care Couple 79

Care Managers 81

Support Networks 83
   Resources for Families 87

Living Options 89
   Aging in Place 89
   Home Sharing 91
   Next Gen Housing 91
   Life Plan Communities 91
   Rehab/Nursing Homes 92
   Village Network 92
   Where to Live: An Exercise 93
   Resources for Housing 94
   Things to Consider: Decision Metrics 96

Managing a Move 97
   Resources for Moving 100
   Our Story: Living in Limbo 102

Acute Incident 109
   Medical Professional Staff Directory 110
   Discharge Orders 111

Taming the Bull 113
   Our Story: Plan C 114
   Our Story: Transfer to a Psychiatric Hospital ... 117
   Our Story: Psych Hospital to Senior Living 120
   "I Want to Go Home" 125
   Our Story: Baby Stalking 128
   Our Story: Safe but Bored 130
   Resources to Enhance the Present 132
   Noted Dementia Care Specialists 134
   Care for the Caregiver / Self-Care and Respite Care 135
   Our Story: Thirty Minutes of Exercise 139

Resources for Caregivers 140
    Movies for Caregivers 141
    Support for Caregivers................................142
    Books for Caregivers 145
    Podcasts for Caregivers 146
        Our Story: Unexpected Angels 146

Approaching the End 151
        Our Story: Suicidal Threats *151*
    Comfort Care: Palliative Care Versus Hospice............ 152
        Our Story: A Stepfather's Last Days.................... *154*
    Death Doulas..155
    Resources for End of Life 156
        Our Story: A Life of Plateaus......................... *157*

Circle of Life.. 159
    Resources for Choosing Insurances 160

You are Not Alone 161

Acknowledgments.................................... 163

INTRODUCTION: THE SILVER TSUNAMI

The silver tsunami of dementia is coming. The oldest baby boomers turned seventy-five in 2021 and their ranks will only get larger.

According to the US Census Bureau, the entire baby boom generation—all 73 million—will be age sixty-five or over by 2030.[2] Their families, including mine, are being thrust into the high-pressure world of eldercare. We are making critical care decisions for parents or grandparents who failed to prepare for the inevitable. In our case, my mother was officially diagnosed with Alzheimer's disease at age seventy-six. In these pages I will share parts of our family story, offered to inform and help you navigate your own family situation. I've created the road map I wish I'd had.

Most currently available books about Alz-heimer's disease and other dementias cover personal stories or clinical care and management protocols. They offer advice on avoiding frustration, help you calmly and productively interact with people with dementia, and stay attentive to, and mindful about, certain behavior patterns.

Diagnosis: Dementia helps you navigate the whole terrain, which encroaches on more and more of your loved one's life and your own. It provides introductory lists of key resources and answers the questions: *Where do I begin? What do I do? How can I get help? What resources are available to me?* It guides you in outlining a plan and assembling a care team of family

---

[2] www.census.gov/library/stories/2019/12/by-2030-all-baby-boomers-will-be-age-65-or-older.html

members, neighbors, friends, community resources, and paid professionals.

Don't do this alone. Communicate with your team and delegate responsibility to manage the legal, financial, and medical aspects of your loved one's situation. Doing so alleviates all those worries, which can overwhelm a caregiver also dealing with the emotional challenge a dementia diagnosis brings. Having a team in place helps deliver the best care possible without overloading one person—you.

Together, you and your team *can* manage the disease with dignity, security, and emotional support. But *Diagnosis: Dementia* doesn't stop there. It also helps you find the help *you* need for your well-being.

There are still many unknowns about Alzheimer's—when it begins, what triggers it, who will get it, how to slow it down. More than a century ago, the disease was discovered and documented, but there still is no cure.

Until a cure is found, we must learn to cope and live with our loved ones in their new reality, on their terms. While science still struggles, countless others have shared stories and developed wonderful methods of interaction, stimulation, and engagement that allow us to enjoy precious time with our loved ones in unprecedented ways. Once you are able to manage the practical problems that cause stress and create anxiety, you also can find peace through simple presence. I will share ways to achieve that peace, too. You can find that peace as long as you accept help.

Nicole J. Smith
Tucson, Arizona
August 2023

**I.
Be Aware**

THE DEMENTIA UMBRELLA

FACT:
Almost 10 percent of Americans ages sixty-five and older have a form of dementia. Another 22 percent have mild cognitive impairment.[3]

Diagnosing dementia is difficult because there are many types and every person, every patient, every situation is unique. Yet the number of families dealing with dementia is prolific.

Dementia is a broad umbrella term used to describe diseases that cause cognitive decline. Alzheimer's disease is the most common type, accounting for between 60 and 80 percent of cases of dementia. It can be broken down into three stages—mild, moderate, and severe memory loss. Sometimes this progression is referred to as early, middle, and late-stage Alzheimer's. The specific traits and behaviors associated with each stage can vary depending on the individual.

The diseases are progressive. Different types are defined by how they affect various parts of the brain. Depending on where the deterioration begins, memory, physical motion, executive function, and personality can change. Some of the more common types of dementia, in addition to Alzheimer's, include Lewy body, vascular dementia, Parkinson's, Huntington's, aphasia, and more. People with Down syndrome have a higher risk of developing dementia. A specific diagnosis is still tough to pinpoint because every brain is unique. Consequently, people

---
[3] www.cuimc.columbia.edu/news/one-10-older-americans-has-dementia

are sometimes diagnosed with a combination of dementias, such as Lewy body and Parkinson's or Alzheimer's and vascular dementia. Brain scans and blood work can provide some clinical clues, but behavior is the basic barometer that signals something is amiss.

A total of 10–11 million Americans are experiencing dementia, according to gerontologist Tam Cummings.[4] Worldwide, more than 55 million people were living with some form of dementia in 2020, according to Alzheimer's Disease International, which reports someone in the world is diagnosed every three seconds.[5]

The number is expected to triple to 131 million by 2050.[6]

---

4   tjpnews.com/the-legacy-offers-staff-training-for-dementia/
5   www.alzint.org/about/dementia-facts-figures/dementia-statistics/
6   www.ncbi.nlm.nih.gov/pmc/articles/PMC6545627/

SIGNS AND SIGNALS

Dementia is an incurable, progressive syndrome that will worsen over time as some of the brain's 100 billion neurons, or nerve cells, are damaged and die.[7]

For every person, dementia progresses differently and on its own timeline. Some sources state subtle changes can begin in the brain ten, even twenty, years prior to symptoms showing up. Brain scans can indicate that plaque buildup exists, but in some people, mysteriously, behavioral changes never materialize.

People who experience an occasional lapse in memory and become concerned can visit their physician or a specialist. Mild Cognitive Impairment (MCI) is the term used to explain occasional and noticeable memory loss that does not significantly affect daily activities.

Signs of early-stage dementia may include losing track of time and/or the season, misplacing items, repeating stories, and forgetting appointments. Short-term memory and communication may become more difficult as the disease progresses. Physical issues become more prominent in the advanced stages.[8]

Yet there are still so many unknowns surrounding dementia: there is no known cause and no definitive treatment. There's also no cure, but there is hope. Awareness, attention, studies, and resources are rising everywhere around the world. All we can do in the present, though, is cope and hope, right from the earliest stages.

---

[7] www.alz.org/alzheimers-dementia/what-is-alzheimers
[8] www.ip-live-in-care.co.uk/7-stages-dementia/

But how can you tell when a loved one is in the early stages of dementia? How can you distinguish MCI from benign forgetfulness? The beginning of dementia is often difficult to detect. You might recognize some of your story in ours.

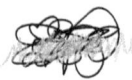

Our Story: The Beginning

Christmas 2017

My mom, sister, and nephews flew from California to New Jersey to spend the holidays with us. We consider our kids spoiled and do not focus on gifts. Years ago we asked the grandparents to stop shopping for the kids, but on Christmas Eve Mom said she'd like to get something small for each kid. I drove her to the local drugstore to buy a few fun stocking stuffers. When we got back to the house, she took them downstairs to the guest room. I gave her paper and other frills to wrap them.

The next morning, Christmas Day, Mom said, "I should have gotten the kids a little something." We reminded her about the drugstore trip. She had forgotten it. We found the untouched bag of gifts she'd purchased in the guest room.

February 2019

Though Mom and her three sisters are scattered around the country, they gather every couple of years to relax, catch up, laugh, and play cards. Nancy, one of the sisters, knew something was amiss when she called my mom shortly after one such reunion: Mom had no recollection of spending a week with her sisters in Florida the previous month. Nancy tried to jog Mom's memory by discussing details of the trip. Details didn't help. Mom always drew a blank.

March 2019

I met my college-age daughter in LA so we could both visit my mom. My nephews, who lived nearby, spent the night with their grandma occasionally. The house had plenty of bedrooms, but the boys liked to drag the "dog bed" cushion and pillows into the family room during sleepovers. Mom and I went out for a casual walk. When we returned, she seemed perplexed at the disarray in the family room.

"Was someone staying here?" she asked. Though I thought her comment strange, I brushed it off.

June 2019

Mom joined us in New Jersey to celebrate my son's high school graduation. As she unzipped her suitcase in the guest room, a pack of cigarettes came flying out and landed across the room. She looked at me.

"Where did that come from?" she asked. I laughed.

"From your suitcase!" I replied.

Mom had smoked years earlier. I knew she was smoking again but I was not overly concerned. She knew the risks and didn't care. Who was I to judge? I also brushed off this absurd occurrence as just weird. I later discovered that smoking can be a significant contributing factor for developing dementia: A 2019 Lancet Commission on dementia prevention ranked smoking as third among nine modifiable risk factors for dementia.[9]

So what was happening in Mom's brain when she forgot about buying the stocking stuffers and the week with her sisters? And what was that like for her?

Think of the frustration you feel when you're looking up something on your computer and get an "ERROR 404: FILE NOT FOUND" message. Behind the scenes the pathway to the website or resource you want is blocked and you can't get to the information you want and need, no matter how much you want to.

The brain of a dementia patient is like a faltering computer with more and more pathways decayed, destroyed, or blocked. Over time, the devastation gets worse. The brain can sometimes create a work-around or generate another pathway to complete a task or retrieve information from another section. It all depends on what parts of the brain are affected and how the disease is advancing. Each person, case, and rate of progression is unique.

---

9 www.alzheimersresearchuk.org/blog/all-you-need-to-know-about-smoking-and-dementia/

Changes in behavior and demeanor can be very subtle. Seniors who live alone probably will not notice or will potentially try to hide any loss in cognitive function. They may not ask for help because they don't want to be a burden on anyone. Couples living together may dismiss cognitive decline in a spouse as typical of the normal aging process or as a minor bout of forgetfulness. Very often people with dementia are quite adept at small talk and polite casual conversation, leaving the impression they are functioning normally. The ability to socially participate reinforces the misconception that any glitch in memory or odd behavior is simply a side effect of aging and not a symptom of something more serious.

The best way to make an initial assessment is to spend consecutive chunks of time together—preferably an overnight stay or several days of visiting—and casually, yet closely, evaluate your parent's cognitive capacity. Then someone should conduct an objective review of your parent's routine, living conditions, medication dosages, general mood, package/postal mail deliveries, financial records, and, if possible, online portals.

Some of the basic questions healthcare professionals initially ask a patient to determine dementia are: What is the name of the current US president? What season are we in now? What day of the week is it? Your parent may pass that kind of test with flying colors and be able to carry on an animated casual conversation, presenting as perfectly "normal" to a nurse or physician who does not know them well.

Many primary care physicians are not thoroughly versed in evaluating dementia, which is a complicated disease. There is no foolproof blueprint to follow though there are some common behavioral patterns that might prompt you to pay more attention: forgetting recent events, being unable to order from a menu or gauge the current season or temperature, asking when lunch will be served fifteen minutes after eating lunch, and repeating questions or stories.

Remember, too, that the typical six-minute appointment does not allow time for a physician to have the kind of meaningful conversation needed to evaluate a patient's history, habits, lifestyle, and preferences. That is why sustained, attentive observation by you, another close family member, or friend can provide a more reliable assessment of whether a loved one should be seen by a trained geriatrician or neurologist.

BEHAVIORAL CHANGES

We all forget things and misplace items. Some forgetfulness *can* be attributed to the normal process of aging, but there is a definite difference between typical versus habitual incidents.

Neuroscientist Lisa Genova, author of the best-selling novel, *Still Alice*, about an Ivy League professor with early-onset Alzheimer's disease, breaks down the difference between typical and habitual: "You'll come to appreciate the clear distinction between normal forgetting (where you parked your car) and forgetting due to Alzheimer's (that you own a car)."[10]

According to Genova, changes in behaviors established over a lifetime can be red flags. Most of the time, family members, friends, and colleagues are the first to notice when we are not behaving as we normally do. Someone with dementia may be challenged when confronted with decision-making or the order of operation for simple tasks, such as picking out clothing for the day or following a familiar recipe. Or they may manifest slight changes in personality, becoming irritable, for instance, or more anxious, or they may exhibit no social filter and speak candidly or inappropriately out of turn in conversation.

These examples can be typical, ordinary behavior patterns for several people we know. The key difference here is if these actions and behaviors are not normal for your parent. The *change* in attitude, demeanor, and behavior could be an indication of dementia.

---
10 www.lisagenova.com/

You know your parent best. Pay particular attention to changes in their habits and behavior patterns involving cooking, driving, medication management, and finances. As you do, bear in mind that certain aspects of a person's daily routine can seem perfectly intact while others can be completely out of character. Note anything that feels or seems out of place and follow up on that instinct with further investigation, conversation, and a little snooping—and, when you feel the time is right, a cognitive assessment.

Remember, even after an assessment and perhaps a prescription, behavioral issues will not simply go away. In fact, they probably will intensify as time goes on.

EVALUATION TOOLS

Getting a memory loss evaluation by a physician provides a snapshot of current memory and thinking capability. That snapshot becomes a baseline that will help measure how your parent's memory loss progresses. It also will determine whether memory changes and challenges are related to dementia, delirium, depression, an adverse medication reaction, or a mix of these factors.

Doctors often don't notice or include memory evaluations in their everyday exam care. Begin educating yourself through videos, blogs, books, and conversations. If you feel in your head, your heart, or your gut that mild cognitive impairment may be an issue, specifically request a cognitive assessment evaluation. You may be referred to a neurologist or not. Be prepared for an evaluation appointment by understanding different tools physicians use. The most common is the Mini-Mental State Examination (MMSE), a popular ten-minute test available in many languages that is adaptable for people with impaired vision.[11]

Other tests assess executive functioning, attention, focus, memory, language, orientation, and the ability to calculate and think conceptually, among other factors. They include the ten-

---

11 www.verywellhealth.com/mini-mental-state-exam-as-an-alzheimers-screening-test-98623

minute Montreal Cognitive Assessment (MoCA)[12] and the Saint Louis University Mental Status Exam (SLUMS), an eleven-question screening questionnaire.[13]

Know that Medicare Part B, which covers outpatient medical coverage, covers a separate visit with your parent's regular doctor, or a specialist, for a full cognitive function assessment. Such a review may establish or confirm a diagnosis and create a care plan.[14]

Another tool or term you may hear is the Global Deterioration Scale (GDS), also known as the Reisberg Scale, after the physician who developed it. The scale begins at 1, which is considered "normal" cognitive ability, and progresses to 7, which indicates severe cognitive decline or severe dementia occurring near the end of life. A score of 4 is considered mild dementia and a signal to keep track of progressive deterioration.[15]

Alzheimer's accounts for 60 to 80 percent of all dementia cases, according to the Centers for Disease Control and Prevention.[16] Whether it's caused by amyloid-beta plaques that trigger tau tangles, or vice versa, is still a matter of debate. Both proteins cumulate in large numbers and clump, disrupting brain functioning[17].

Those with early-onset Alzheimer's, which causes behavioral issues before age sixty-five, tend to have what is called the common form of the disease, which progresses much the same way it does in older patients. Genetic, or familial, Alzheimer's, is rare. Those who have it start showing symptoms in their thirties, forties, or fifties, according to Johns Hopkins Medicine, which reports that only a few hundred people have genes that directly cause the disease.[18]

---

12 mocacognition.com
13 www.slu.edu/medicine/internal-medicine/geriatric-medicine/aging-successfully/assessment-tools/mental-status-exam.php
14 www.medicare.gov/coverage/cognitive-assessment-care-plan-services
15 geriatrictoolkit.missouri.edu/cog/Global-Deterioration-Scale.pdf
16 www.cdc.gov/aging/dementia/index.html
17 www.nia.nih.gov/health/what-happens-brain-alzheimers-disease
18 www.hopkinsmedicine.org/health/conditions-and-diseases/alzheimers-disease/earlyonset-alzheimer-disease

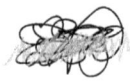

Our Story: Getting Tested

During their frequent phone calls, Mom complained to her sister, Nancy, an RN for more than fifty years, about random aches and pains. She said she'd visited her primary physician several times but never came away with a clear diagnosis.

Over time Nurse Nancy flew from the East Coast to LA to accompany Mom to some diagnostic doctor appointments. As Mom's designated medical power of attorney, Nancy also began to monitor mom's healthcare portal more closely. A medical power of attorney is separate from a financial power of attorney. Both are critical to have in place and discussed later in the book.

Mom's medical records revealed that her primary care physician had ordered lab work, an MRI, and a neurologist appointment months earlier. Mom had never followed through on any of them. Had she been in denial? During this time she changed doctors because she wanted a different opinion.

While she was in California, Nancy scheduled the various tests and accompanied Mom to some of them. After Nancy flew home, Mom's youngest daughter, who lived locally, was available to help with the other appointments.

March 17, 2020

Nancy requested that I fly out from the East Coast to accompany Mom to her first appointment with the neurologist, Dr. Kurz, who had specifically requested that a family member be present for the evaluation. COVID-19 was just ramping up and authorities were still uncertain about how bad it really was and whether it would disappear in a couple of weeks. I flew to California.

Finally, the moment of truth arrived. Mom and I exchanged pleasantries with the neurologist. She asked Mom the basic questions about diet, exercise, and sleep. She also asked Mom if she smoked.

"Yes, I smoke, but I don't inhale," Mom replied. The classic Bill Clinton defense! She was completely serious. I burst out laughing. The doctor smirked. Already annoyed at my presence and the fact we were even at the appointment, my mom dismissed me shortly thereafter. I didn't like that. However, I respected the doctor's need to ensure her patient was calm and comfortable so she could conduct a thorough, accurate assessment.

The neurologist was able to reach Nancy by phone on the opposite coast and got the family input she needed. Mom was more comfortable with that approach as I sat, stewing, in the waiting room. I'd flown cross-country in the midst of global uncertainty, just to be booted out five minutes into the meeting.

After leaving that appointment, Mom could not remember where we'd parked the car. Of course that can happen to anyone on a strange campus of buildings and parking decks, all jumbled together. We found the car and, as we headed home, decided to stop at the Starbucks in her neighborhood. She had been to that Starbucks dozens of times. It was a ten-minute walk from her house. When I parked in a lot one block away, Mom freaked out and refused to walk anywhere because she couldn't see the building's awning. She didn't believe me when I told her the coffee shop was on the next block. We had to return to the car and park directly across the street from Starbucks. Very odd.

As the world shut down, I flew home. I would have brought her back to New Jersey with me if I had known we were going into lockdown. But who knew? It would have been a tough sell, anyway, to get her to leave her beloved bright and sunny LA.

In isolation she began smoking more. She hadn't smoked for years but began again to be "closer to Bert," my stepfather who had passed away from cancer in 2002. He'd been a heavy smoker. Mom was just done with life and ready to be gone and join Bert.

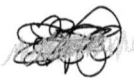

Our Story: COVID-19

The extended isolation probably contributed to the progression of Mom's disease. Lack of socialization is of concern for aging adults, especially those with mild cognitive impairment.

I called her almost daily during COVID-19. She was very lonely. She said she spent her time working in the yard and taking walks. I had no reason to disbelieve her. She was perfectly cordial talking on the phone and seemed to be holding her own, as we all tried to do during lockdown. Not until I finally flew out to spend significant time with her did I notice all was not as it seemed. It is easy to be immersed in our own lives and assured that all is well. To make things worse, many parents do not want to be a burden and intentionally discourage relatives from visiting and discovering the layers of dust on the furniture, the moldy food in the fridge, mobility issues, and other subtle signs of decline.

When COVID-19 hit my mother was totally alone indefinitely. Her daughter and grandkids who lived locally stopped visiting her. The fear and uncertainty of the potentially deadly and unknown virus spreading across the globe affected everyone. Mom masked up and ventured out every couple of weeks to get groceries. It was the highlight of her existence to be among humans again, if only briefly, as one of her 2021 journal entries clearly showed:

Sunday, August 29, 2021

Having a very difficult time thinking! I am in a fog, can't figure out what's happening to my mind. I'm scared and very confused!

It's an empty, lonely time. I do know that I'm okay when I'm around others—but that's not something that happens a lot.

Nicole's visit last week was helpful! I must find a way to be around others on a regular basis. It helps my brain function. Call Sherry and set a date with her. Lisa will be back home soon—go spend time with her! Visit Doris weekly!

Mom managed to keep a routine of doing puzzles, listening to music, and hanging out on the porch to watch the many passersby. Her house sat on a busy through street, one block removed from the main artery into the neighborhood on the hill. The location was perfect for people watching. Walkers, joggers, and baby strollers frequently paraded by in the sunny SoCal weather at all hours of the day. "The singing walker" sang loudly and proudly during her daily stroll.

Our phone conversations were brief, as there wasn't any news to share. I had a house full of kids again and talked about the daily routine of cooking and repeating fifth grade with my youngest, who would frequently wander away from the screen if I wasn't physically present to ensure he paid attention.

I invited and encouraged Mom to join us on the East Coast and become part of our "bubble." She appreciated the offer but refused to get on a plane or accept our invitation to fly out and drive her back. She wanted to stay in the sunshine and her familiar surroundings. So, like most of the world, she remained completely isolated for months.

In 2021 Nancy and I did tag team cross-country flights to stay with Mom and get ahead of sorting through her house because we knew it had to be sold. We didn't have much success. My mother sat me down daily and, in her domineering way, emphatically explained how she was completely in control and perfectly capable of staying in her home.

Yet there was constant paranoia. She feared that Nancy and I were talking with her doctors behind her back and plotting to put her away when, in her view, she was managing fine on her own. She was alternately irate at us, calling one of us untrustworthy while designating the other as the "only one I can trust." The roles continually rotated.

"You refuse to believe anything you don't want to believe as true," I once told her. "You cannot sustain the current financial situation in this house."

The statement did not break her stride. She declared that she journaled extensively and thus knew when we were not telling her the truth. She said she could check her journals for accuracy on any situation because she recorded her accounts as they happened. And so the struggle continued between her desperate attempt to retain control and our frustration in figuring out how to convince her it was time to move.

COOKING

Unattended cooking is by far the leading factor in most kitchen fires. Cooking causes 49 percent of reported home fires in the US.[19] Stories about an unattended, forgotten pot on the stove are commonly told in caregiver circles and identified as a sign of something being amiss. Some families simply have the gas turned off in the home to avoid a cooking calamity.

This excerpt from a Massachusetts newspaper lays out the relationship between dementia and house fires from a fire prevention point of view:

> Fire professionals have identified four types of fire risk for individuals living with Alzheimer's disease, other dementias, and memory loss. The first is related to a person's past role or actions. Examples include someone who has always smoked in bed or a retired electrician who continues to do repairs around the house. The second risk involves using appliances inappropriately. Putting metal trays in the microwave or heating a glass dish directly on the stove are common problems in this category. The third risk is directly related to memory loss and may involve forgetting to turn off the gas on the stove, a space heater, or accidentally leaving food in a hot oven. The fourth risk is related to the individual's home environment and includes overloaded outlets, clutter, and leaving flammable items too close to a heat source.[20]

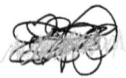

Our Story: Food

My mother rarely cooked. I grew up in the '70s on SpaghettiOs, TV dinners, and sugared cereals. Fortunately, we did not have to worry about her leaving the stove on. She primarily ate iceberg lettuce with carrots, rotisserie chicken wrapped in tortillas (with a little mayonnaise for a tangy taste), blueberries, yogurt, and Ritz

---

19 www.nfpa.org/-/media/Files/News-and-Research/Fire-statistics-and-reports/US-Fire-Problem/Fire-causes/oscooking.pdf

20 thewestfieldnews.com/retire-the-fire-dementia-memory-loss-and-fire-safety-2/

crackers. Not an ideal varied diet, but no cooking required. The fact that Mom bought the same things over and over, regardless of whether she had depleted her existing supply, was another red flag if we had paid attention. She had several containers of rotting blueberries stacked in the fridge but bought a new batch each time because the routine purchases were familiar to her waning brain.

DRIVING

Driving is one of the de facto definitions of independence. For a teenager, it is an anxiously anticipated milestone to freedom, but for an older person who stops driving, it can mean the loss of freedom—yet another blow to the ego. Some neighborhoods and communities offer bus routes that shuttle seniors to appointments and grocery shopping. Modern apps offer ride services and enable grocery delivery options, too, but the experience is not the same and many seniors resist when it's suggested they should give up their license.

Yet not driving is often a good idea. AAA reports that, for the first time in history, older people should plan for their so-called "driving retirement." Why? Seniors are outliving their ability to drive safely by an average of seven to ten years. Statistics back up this idea: seniors have the second highest crash death rate per mile driven, outpaced only by teenagers.[21]

If you need help or proof that your parent is no longer driving at their best, or even unsafely, you can reach out to AAA[22] or AARP[23] for professional and self-rated driving skills evaluation tests and senior driver safety courses.

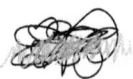

Our Story: Driving Miss Crazy

Mom had always been an aggressive driver and was usually on the go. She kept her car immaculate and loved the power of independence it afforded her. As her memory faded, she relied

---
21 exchange.aaa.com/safety/senior-driver-safety-mobility/
22 exchange.aaa.com/safety/senior-driver-safety-mobility/evaluate-your-driving-ability/
23 campaigns.aarp.org/driversafetycourse/

on SIRI for navigation. Even with SIRI helping, she got confused about directions and often was late to meet people or was gone for hours. She always found her way home, eventually. She covered her mistakes by claiming she just enjoyed driving around, killing time while getting lost among the beautiful LA mountains.

We were nervous about her driving and we knew preventing her from doing so would mean fighting an extremely difficult battle. So we were relieved to be able to blame the state of California for taking her keys away: California law requires a physician to notify the Division of Motor Vehicles (DMV) about a dementia diagnosis.

Mom was livid. She frequently referred to a notation her primary care physician had made in her online medical portal two years earlier: it stated she was "OK to drive." Mom had a standard set of rote, rehearsed soliloquies she repeated often to convince herself and others of her competency and control. "OK to drive" became one of her new "Mom mantras," which she added to her litany of loops.

She even declared that if her license was revoked, she would kill herself. She repeated the threat so frequently that Nancy scheduled a mental health assessment with Mom's physician. Nancy made the cross-country trek again to accompany Mom to that appointment and more.

Mom received letters from the DMV outlining various stages of review required before her license could be reinstated. She had to have a phone interview with the DMV, followed by a visit to the office to complete her vision and written exams. Nancy was in LA to facilitate these meetings and the process.

During the initial phone interview with the DMV, Mom explained she didn't need to know how to get anywhere because SIRI always got her where she needed to be. Nancy accompanied Mom to the DMV for the next round, the vision and written tests. Nancy observed Mom taking the vision test, reporting it was somewhat comical to watch. Somehow Mom passed that round. She proceeded to another area, monitored by a proctor, to take the written test. Unaware of the "NO PHONES" signs displayed everywhere, she pulled her phone out of her purse to answer an incoming call while she was testing. She was promptly ordered to leave without finishing the test.

A week later, a letter arrived from the DMV to notify Mom that, effective September 8, 2021, her privilege to operate a motor vehicle was withdrawn because her written test results were unsatisfactory. She refused to accept this outcome, destroyed the letter, and hid subsequent DMV letters that arrived in the mail. She continued to obsess over the testing procedure and called the DMV repeatedly to escalate her complaint. Each time they referred her to their driver safety program and gave her the phone number to call that department.

Mom wrote notes to herself on scraps of paper, Sticky Notes, and random envelopes: "My Dr. did not talk to me about No driving … get a second opinion on my rights … call Volvo for keys—where are they?" Nancy had taken her car keys. Nancy was Mom's big sister, so she could get away with doing some things the rest of us couldn't.

Still, Mom kept obsessing over the insult of losing her license and wrote more notes: "Call lawyer, remove Nancy from my list … message her for being awful."

I arrived back in LA to relieve Nancy and attempted to convince Mom to go through closets to prepare for an eventual move. My sister joined us for dinner, so the three of us could collectively meet in person to decide what to do about moving Mom. We did not include Mom in the meeting, but she lurked outside the room in anger. We didn't want her derailing the meeting with more Mom mantras. Things had been getting messy with the plan to move her. She was becoming more belligerent. Mom was determined to be disruptive so we decided to adjourn and try again another time. My sister went home and Mom retreated to her room, per her usual routine. Nancy and I settled in for the night in our respective bedrooms to read.

Around 9 p.m. I wandered out of my room and noticed Mom's bedroom door was open. I peeked in to check on her, but she was not there. She was not anywhere in the house. I summoned Nancy. We were worried. Nancy still had the car keys, so we figured Mom could not have ventured too far on foot. We didn't know what time she had left the house. All we knew was her state of mind: rageful and defiant. I called her cell but got no answer. Nancy took off in the car to look for her while I stayed back at the house in case Mom returned.

Nancy returned thirty minutes later—without Mom. We were discussing our next plan of action when Mom came walking up the driveway. She was still angry and agitated but safe and home. We all went to bed.

After that incident, we set up tracking on Mom's phone, linked to mine, in case she decided to go wandering off again. She did.

A few days later Nancy was to take an early morning flight home. I was up and ready to drive her to the airport in Mom's car when Mom came downstairs, frantic and screaming that someone had stolen her driver's license. She kept accusing us of going through her things and taking it. Mom reasoned that, regardless of what the DMV dictated, she still had possession of her driver's license, so she was "OK to drive."

Nancy and I explained that we had not taken anything and suggested she look through her purse again. The DMV drama was still in full swing. Nancy gave me both sets of car keys and instructed me to always keep them on my person. As Nancy and I left for the airport, Mom went back upstairs to rummage through her documents.

A couple of days later, I drove Mom to the DMV because she insisted that she had an appointment to retest and reinstate her license. I doubted this was true but humored her because it allowed her to assume a sense of control and it gave us something to do. I was in survival mode.

When we arrived at the DMV, Mom told me to wait in the parking lot while she took care of this misunderstanding. Fifteen minutes later, she returned with another referral to the driver safety program and the phone number.

We stopped at the local grocery store to get a few things. She was following me with the cart. I stopped to check out the meat section. When I turned around, she was gone! I didn't know much about dementia, but I knew some people tended to wander off. All I could think was, *I lost her? How could I lose her in the grocery store?* I panicked. I didn't think she was that far gone yet. Thankfully, I found her quickly. She had intentionally ditched me to buy cigarettes. She was still trying to deceive me about her little habit, even though I sat with her while she openly smoked on the patio at home. I was in over my head.

Despite Mom's protests, I was determined to go through the house to identify long-forgotten items to donate. I kept flying across the country so I was intent on being productive while I was there, even if it was slow going and I had to be sneaky about it.

One morning I even snuck out and drove to a local charity to donate business clothes from one of the closets. I made several clandestine donation trips when Mom was still asleep. Sometimes I made up an excuse to go out and use the car, careful to conceal any contraband donations in the trunk.

Though Mom spewed a diatribe of denial at us, she knew something was wonky with her brain. Her prolific random written notes revealed her frustration and fear: "What else do I need to do? Don't want to screw something up in this process of selling house … find someone to help sort out and sell all of my stuff. I really can't do that alone."

Mom expressed her concerns and vulnerability whenever we spoke on the phone long-distance, but soon after I arrived in person to help execute her plan, she pulled a complete reversal. She assumed a calm demeanor of superiority and launched into yet another Mom mantra explanation about how she intended to remain in her house, had everything under control, and was perfectly capable of managing her life on her own.

"Thank you for coming," she told me. "I am so glad you are here. Now please change your flight and leave."

Meanwhile, she continued to ruminate over the DMV, the car, the keys. One day I took off for a quick jog to clear my head. When I returned, I could tell she had gone through my bags and belongings, looking for the keys while I was out. I did not keep them on my person and had them well hidden under a cushion and on a random closet shelf. We fought all day.

Eventually, she got extremely enraged and took off on foot to the grocery store. Once she got to the Ralph's grocery store

DIAGNOSIS: DEMENTIA—21

about a mile away, she called my brother-in-law and asked him to pick her up, admitting she wasn't sure where she was. She asked a random stranger to tell her which street they were on so my brother-in-law could pick her up. This was the same Ralph's we had walked to every day during my visits, the one where she had often shopped since she'd moved to LA more than twenty years earlier.

My brother-in-law said he was working and would break away if he could. She told him not to call me or tell me about the call. Of course, he called me immediately.

I drove the car around the neighborhood and found her walking back home. Maybe she used her phone to navigate back or returned to a familiar pathway in her brain. We had dinner plans with my brother-in-law that night. I knew I had to spend some time with rational humans for a reprieve. Nancy had only been gone two days and I was already losing my mind being alone with Mom. She refused to go to dinner with me. I went anyway. I figured that with me out of the house, she would calm down and have some peace. When I returned later that night, she was holed up in her room.

The next day I continued to sort through cupboards and closets. I pulled more than fifty binders of archaic training materials from the family room cabinets to recycle the paper and trash the binders. As I took a break to log into a Zoom call, I watched as Mom swooped in and returned every binder back to the cabinet shelves. Argh! She told me to change my flight and leave her house.

I reminded her that she had a hair appointment that afternoon. She refused to believe I knew what time the appointment was, so she kept calling the salon to confirm. She had a habit of deleting any text messages about appointments. I dropped her at the salon and went to meet an elder law attorney.

A couple of hours later, I pulled up in front of the salon and found easy parking right outside the giant sidewalk window where Mom was sitting with her stylist. He looked out and waved and mentioned I was outside. Mom looked out.

"That's not my car," she said.

22—DIAGNOSIS: DEMENTIA

"Your daughter is driving it," he said, "so it is your car."

After the appointment we decided to stop at the grocery store. Mom criticized my driving and complained about not being able to drive "my own damn car." As we pulled into the parking space, she reached across and tried to yank the key out of the dash before the car had fully stopped! I screamed, put the car in park, and took the key. She punched me in the arm. I yelled at her, stormed out of the car, and went into the store to call Nancy. I was extremely flustered.

I bought beer and ice cream and returned to the car to find Mom calmly waiting. I drove home, opened a beer, and ignored her for the rest of the evening.

Mom grew angrier by the day. She kept telling me to leave. I had planned to stay another week and spend Thanksgiving with her, so she wouldn't be lonely. I tried to avoid her, keep a low profile, and stay out of her way. I was exhausted. She continued to seek me out and badger me with her Mom mantras. I decided to grant her wish for me to exit the premises. When she went out for a walk, I packed up my stuff and drove her car to my sister's condo. We decided the car would be safe in the condo parking garage for the time being. I changed my flight and flew back to New Jersey for Thanksgiving. My kids were happy I was home to cook! Mom left me a voice mail.

"Are you coming back?" she asked.

I did not respond.

Soon Mom figured out her car was gone and guessed it was probably with my sister and her boys. She called all of them, repeatedly demanding they bring the car back. My sister drove the car back over to Mom's house and left it there but she kept all the car keys.

A couple of days later, we got a call from one of Mom's neighbors. She wanted to let us know a locksmith van was parked outside Mom's house. Mom had paid $1,400 to have new keys made and then took off in the car to run errands. The fact that she was driving again, illegally, caused great concern, and would lead to even more problems later because of the locksmith charge on her credit card.

Nancy and I called my sister to ask her to take the car and keep it away from Mom. She agreed but called the police to ask their advice on how to handle the situation. They informed her that, even though Mom's license had been suspended by the State of California, her car was considered personal property. If it was taken without Mom's permission and reported stolen, my sister would be held accountable and possibly arrested! Unbelievable.

We were pretty sure Mom would not hesitate to report it stolen and my sister didn't want to risk going to jail. That night she left the car with Mom. A couple of days later, Mom drove the car—and lost it. We received several worried texts from neighbors: Mom had lost her keys while at the grocery store where she happened to bump into a neighbor, who took her home.

Mom then got the extra set of new keys from the house and wandered the neighborhood, searching for someone else to take her back to the parking lot to retrieve her car. One couple agreed to help her. They all went together. The couple drove the car home for her. The wife, who happened to be a psychotherapist, handled the situation with utmost care. The neighbors were already somewhat aware of Mom's cognitive challenges and our desperate attempts to get help. They were gracious in communicating with us, but they did not feel comfortable taking her keys away.

The entire scenario repeated itself two weeks later: Mom drove to the grocery store. After shopping, she could not locate her car in the parking lot. Immediately, she assumed it had been stolen. Again, she happened to see a neighbor and asked her to help look for the car. When they could not find it, the neighbor drove her home.

Mom called the police and reported the car stolen. My sister still had the original sets of keys, so she drove over to the grocery store. The car was there in the parking lot, right where Mom had left it. My sister drove the car back to her condo and parked it under the building, out of sight.

Mom got busy filing the report, notifying her insurance company, and arranging for a rental car. It gave her something to focus on, even though the claim was false. I arrived back in LA the next day and set the record straight with the police and the insurance company before any claims were processed.

My sister eventually located the mental health person within the police department to explain our situation. They agreed the car could and should remain parked and "stolen." Mom would not drive her car again, but she would continue to drive us crazy!

MEDICATION MANAGEMENT

Managing meds is critical. Organized pillboxes may help some people, but human oversight is best. Many people see multiple specialists for myriad ailments and conditions. One specialist may prescribe something that a second specialist is unaware of. How might those two prescriptions interact? Medicine has become highly specialized and a lack of communication and review can be concerning.

While pharmacy commercials advertise how their customer care systems monitor information and prevent dangerous combinations, it's best to double-check your loved one's meds. You or a care manager should conduct a detailed review of all meds, including over-the-counter pills, vitamins, and supplements.

Be aware of any possible side effects and watch for them. Someone should be spending time with your loved one to monitor any changes in behavior when prescriptions are added and/or dosages modified.

Remember that sometimes prescriptions are added when a person is admitted to the hospital after an acute episode or fall. Sometimes these prescriptions, which may no longer be necessary, follow the patient home. To ensure this doesn't happen to your loved one, Jean Ross, a nurse and family caregiver advocate, urges caregivers to speak up and request a "medication reconciliation," which, she says, health professionals are required to conduct after any transition.

Additionally, Ross urges caregivers to check the Beers Criteria List, which identifies common and potentially inappropriate medications for older adults.[24] Nine types are most common. Some may be okay for an older person to take in certain circumstances,

---
24 my.clevelandclinic.org/health/articles/24946-beers-criteria

according to Ross, who added that, nevertheless, the list should be consulted.

More than 40 percent of Americans age sixty-five and older take at least five medications, known as "polypharmacy." The number, according to a 2020 Lown Institute report, reflects a 200 percent increase over the past twenty years.[25]

In his best-selling book, *Being Mortal*, Atul Gawande, surgeon and public health researcher, writes that there are three primary risk factors for the elderly falling: poor balance, muscle weakness, and taking more than four prescription medications.

"Elderly people without these risk factors have a 12 percent chance of falling in a year," Gawande writes. "Those with all three risk factors have almost a 100 percent chance."

There's more: an older adult who takes at least five meds has a 50 percent chance of being hospitalized due to a negative drug reaction. For dementia patients, overmedication can be even more risky, according to DailyCaring.com, an online magazine for family caregivers.[26] In fact, some meds, prescription and over-the-counter, can actually make dementia worse.

A case in point is diphenhydramine, a common over-the-counter option to alleviate allergy symptoms. Some know it by its common brand name, Benadryl. Diphenhydramine limits an important brain chemical, acetylcholine, a neurotransmitter used for learning, memory, and muscle functions. Our bodies naturally produce less acetylcholine as we age. Actively blocking it with drugs makes it all the more difficult for the brain to deliver instructions—the last thing a dementia patient needs. Sometimes the drug can even bring about dementia-like symptoms in older adults who don't have dementia.[27]

Other drugs for dementia patients to avoid include benzodiazepine, corticosteroids, and, sometimes, beta-blockers, statins, and, temporarily, chemo drugs.[28]

---

25 www.nextavenue.org/medication-overload-growing-problem/
26 dailycaring.com/medications-worsen-dementia-and-increase-dementia-risk-anticholinergics/
27 dailycaring.com/overmedication-worsens-dementia-how-to-avoid-medication-problems-geriatric-academy/
28 www.healthline.com/health/dementia/dementia-medications-to-avoid#meds-associated-with-dementia

If you feel your loved one may need to stop taking some potentially unnecessary med, consider "deprescribing," a process that promotes reducing or stopping medications that may no longer be beneficial or may even be detrimental.[29] The goal of deprescribing is to improve quality of life.

Managing the meds along with making doctor appointments, shopping, cleaning, running errands, and worrying is overwhelming. Documenting everything as it happens, saving receipts to manage the timeline, and keeping things data-driven and organized can help—if you force yourself into the habit of doing so. Many families have a master binder where they keep everything.

Caregivers looking for a secure digital place to invite in other family or support professionals can utilize apps or features on phones to keep track of everything. One such app is Primary Record, cofounded by Ross and her neighbor, a caregiver and technologist. Primary Record helps your family members and healthcare team easily share and manage your loved one's medical information and health stories by storing them in one place.[30]

Bottom line, meds should be monitored regularly for those experiencing memory loss, especially after an incident, a visit to a new doctor, or a change in health status. Make a point of conducting a comprehensive review periodically, in your spare time!

Our Story: Managing Meds

The neurologist had prescribed Aricept for Mom upon her initial diagnosis. Mom had the prescription and took it for a month while Nancy was there to remind her. Then she stopped, as it was outside her normal routine. She lived alone, so nobody was there to remind her of the change or ensure that she took it. Sometimes she remembered what meds she was on; other times she did not.

---

29 deprescribing.org/
30 www.primaryrecord.com/about/

October 20, 2021

We finally arrived at the day of the follow-up appointment with Dr. Kurz, the neurologist—the primary reason for my visit. Flash back to March 17, 2020, when I first flew out to accompany Mom to an appointment with Dr. Kurz as COVID-19 was threatening to shut down the country and the world.

That time she had gone willingly. This time would be a challenge because she had been cursing Dr. Kurz ever since the Alzheimer's diagnosis triggered her driver's license suspension.

Mom often deleted things from her phone that she didn't want to deal with or perceived as a scam. She got frequent text messages from the medical system confirming an upcoming appointment, which she promptly deleted every time. The doctor gave Nancy the number for her office manager so we could communicate directly to assure them we would absolutely be at the appointment and to make sure the system notes reflected that fact. Here's how it worked: The automated appointment system sent Mom a text. She declined/canceled the appointment. We called the office manager and asked them to reinstate the appointment. They never figured out how to stop the notifications or else they couldn't because of privacy regulations. Who knows? This cycle happened at least four times leading up to the October appointment.

Another challenge was creating a ruse to get Mom to go to the medical center. She was due for her COVID-19 booster, so I went with that. She was confused and didn't understand why she had to go to the medical center when the booster was available at every corner drugstore. I told her it was "specific to her health plan." After some coaxing she got in the car, but we were late. I was terrified, exhausted, and scrambling.

After several discussions with our elder law attorney, we learned that to manifest the move for Mom we needed to establish incapacity. All of Mom's assets were in a trust she had established years earlier. Estate planning in every state is different, depending on probate law. Mom was the grantor and trustee of her own trust, but her document included a somewhat standard clause stating that control of the assets would be passed to a successor trustee (me) if she was declared incapacitated. Two licensed physicians had to independently declare Mom incapacitated. As you can imagine, there is exposure for abuse. Therefore, many physicians are reluctant to get involved in legal matters.

Nevertheless, we needed signed letters from the doctors declaring incapacity to invoke the terms of the trust. Nancy had prepared a document laying out Mom's recent fall, her errant behavior, her defiance, and our desperation to find a safe place for her. Her written narrative, including a chart, reflected all our concerns:

BEHAVIORAL CHANGES / CONCERNS

- Rarely cleaning house (huge change)
- Memories lost/no recollection:
  - 1 month after weeklong sister reunion
  - 2 weeks after granddaughter visit
  - 2 days after dinner with friends
- Unable to navigate unfamiliar environments
- Unable to follow movie plots/news reports
- Withdrawal from friends/outings
- Rages/rants regarding driver license
- Pacing/agitation/shouting
- Statements of self-harm:
  - "I'm not going to be here"
  - "I could drive off a high ridge road nearby"
  - "There are ways to kill myself"
  - "I should have the right to die"
  - "If that is the case, I know what I will do"

SAFETY AND FINANCIAL

- Smoking 1–2 packs per day
- Declaration of intent to drive without valid driver's license. Obsessed with DMV letters and appointments. Disposed of letters revoking her license.
- Losing cards: driver's license, Medicare, legal docs
- Accuses family members of taking docs/cards
- Fell down main staircase at home twice
- Paid insurance bill twice
- Cancels doctor appointments
- Frequent calls to credit card customer service to refute charges because she doesn't recall making them. Defiant demands for representative to "escalate the call" to upper management to resolve her problems.

I printed out Nancy's letter, added my own written notes, and enclosed it in an envelope. We hoped Dr. Kurz would be able to read the letter before Mom's appointment to emphasize our dire situation.

We checked in at the desk, Mom announcing she was there to receive her COVID-19 booster shot. The receptionist looked confused. I was standing behind Mom and emphatically nodded affirmation so she would go along with our plan. She did. When Mom turned away, I thrust the envelope labeled "Dr. Kurz" at the receptionist with a pleading look. She understood.

Mom was perturbed and grumbling that this was ridiculous for an appointment for a booster shot. I grabbed a magazine and pretended to read so I could feign ignorance.

A nurse invited us into the back area for a blood pressure check. Mom again expressed her discontent about the booster process. The nurse started to question and clarify but thankfully stopped when she saw my facial expression.

We proceeded down the hall and into Dr. Kurz's office. She welcomed Mom, who just went with it and acted like she wasn't surprised to see the doctor again. I figured I would have hell to pay from Mom after this appointment, but at least we'd made it.

We chatted before Dr. Kurz put Mom through some assessments. Mom was fine making small talk, but she could not identify what day of the week it was or what season we were in. Most of the questions confused her. She carried on, mostly calm, until she broke down slightly at one point.

"This is hard to endure," she said. Dr. Kurz was empathetic.

"Tell me the medications you're on now," she said to Mom.

"The only thing I ever took is a sleeping pill," Mom replied. She had never taken sleeping pills that I was aware of. She regularly took a few basic scripts for relatively minor, manageable conditions, but she could not name any of them. We were fairly certain she was still taking them because they were part of her routine.

I was relieved to see that the letter I had passed to the receptionist was on Dr. Kurz's desk, tucked near the wall next to her computer screen. Dr. Kurz read through it while Mom was taking a timed assessment on paper. When both were finished, Dr. Kurz reiterated her concern that Mom should not continue to live alone.

Mom blamed everything on the pandemic. Dr. Kurz suggested she see a psychologist and consider moving into a senior facility. Mom went along with the suggestions, as she always did, to appear cooperative. In actuality, she had no intention of relinquishing her independence or control.

We thanked Dr. Kurz and left. I hoped we had sufficiently demonstrated our desperation.

I waited for the backlash from Mom for tricking her. There was none. She had forgotten why we came in the first place. As luck would have it, they were running a COVID-19 clinic in the building that morning and she was able to get her booster!

On the way home we went to the pharmacy to get her Aricept. When we chatted over coffee, Mom had no recollection of visiting Dr. Kurz that morning.

In 2022, toward the end of our horrendous episode with moving Mom, a neighbor shared that she had suspected Mom was having issues when she couldn't remember the rules for mah-jongg. The neighbor had noticed this a couple of *years* before the rest of us did. Mom had never been a big fan of games other than playing cards, so when we discovered she had quit playing mah-jongg with the neighbors, we had just figured she'd grown tired of it.

If we had been paying attention, we would have picked up on her withdrawal from one of her only outlets for socialization. She was simply too embarrassed to continue going, even though the neighbors were more than accommodating and understanding. They didn't express their concerns to the family because they did not know us that well. Strangers certainly don't insert themselves into others' delicate medical matters. We had missed many of the signs because we were visiting sporadically and Mom was meticulous about hiding her limitations from us.

It is often those closest to us—family members, coworkers, neighbors—who first notice a change in normal behavior or memory lapses.

FINANCES

Sometimes simply sifting through your parent's mail can help you discover if they are slipping with money management. Late notices from utility companies may be piling up. Random packages and bills from unfamiliar online ordering establishments could be a sign your parent is lonely, making them more likely to chat with solicitors and purchase unnecessary items. Fraud is a concern, too. Grifters are crafty with their schemes. Combing through the mail is one way to flush them out.

Exercise discretion when going through your parent's mail, even if it is to protect them. Paranoia can be a prominent problem with those who suffer from dementia. Mom was exceptionally paranoid about everything we did or said. She was so desperate to hide her shortcomings, she went to great lengths to turn the shame and blame on me or Nancy or whoever was around for doubting her, even though we were trying to help.

Many adults have embraced the automation of bill paying. For others, though, it remains a critical, routine, and basic task. Paying attention to your parent's incoming mail or messages on an answering machine may indicate whether paying bills has become a problem. Are there past due notices? Are creditors leaving multiple messages? These kinds of clues can help you open a conversation about personal finance matters—a tough subject even in the closest of families. The American Association of Daily Money Managers certifies individuals who can help with the tedious process of bill paying and keeping papers organized.[31] For those who are overwhelmed or caregiving from a distance, a money manager can offer peace of mind for one piece of the financial puzzle.

Forbes magazine offers two more caveats to watch for: evidence of excessive charitable giving and/or any new "friend" in your parent's life who seems overly interested in their affairs.[32]

I listened to an interview with a New Jersey elder law attorney who had worked to rescue a client's house from foreclosure. His client was a woman in her eighties, living alone, who had missed several quarterly property tax payments. There are legitimate businesses that capitalize on these lapses and can legally take title to a person's home if the homeowner is unable to foot the bill for any past due tax payments.

A business had in fact made the octogenarian's payments in the amount of about $12,000 and was now preparing to foreclose on the property and seize her only asset, her home, valued at $700,000. Fortunately, a family member going through her mail realized something was up and contacted this attorney, who was able to restore title and ownership to the elderly woman, but not until she paid the $12,000 in taxes owed on the property, plus another $10,000 to cover the court costs associated with clearing up the legal mess. Capture the mail!

---

31 secure.aadmm.com/
32 www.forbes.com/sites/carolynrosenblatt/2015/12/11/three-warning-signs-your-aging-parent-needs-help-handling-finances

Our Story: Legal Documents

August 2021

Mom and I started going through some papers in her office. I happened upon some legal documents and realized she had recently changed her will again; a neighbor couple had signed as witnesses. I was a little unnerved.

In 2019 Nancy had spent weeks working with Mom to get her legal documents in order. Writing family members in and out of a will when there's a family feud is not uncommon, but with Mom's Alzheimer's diagnosis, coupled with her paranoia, any changes were a concern. Handling cognition can be a gray area, legally speaking, but we knew we didn't need this additional uncertainty as we were planning to move her.

When Mom left with the car to run an errand, I saw my chance to capture and copy the will and trust documents before my initial meeting with the elder law attorney. I was paranoid she would discover them missing if I took the originals, so I hoofed it to the neighborhood library to make copies. I could have called an Uber, but I was wound tight with nervous energy I needed to discharge. So I threw the documents in a bag over my shoulder and briskly walked the mile and a half in the scorching summer heat. The library was well equipped with an electronic scanning system that made paper copies and even enabled me to email them to myself.

I was clumsy and disorganized as I unclipped, stacked, and fed the papers through the machine, trying not to expose my daughterly guilt. The librarian was helpful and polite although I felt like a crazed lunatic on a spy mission. The green flash sliding under the glass to the whir of gears mimicked the anxious buzz in my brain.

Feelings of betrayal, defiance, and disobe-dience swelled inside me as perspiration seeped out of every pore. I did not feel comfortable rummaging through my mother's private papers, but we were desperate to save her from herself. I had been named in several places in the trust documents and had received copies when she first completed them, but we had no idea how many times she had changed the papers since then. And if we were to manage her move and care legally, we had to know who controlled what. I didn't like sneaking around, but her paranoia prevented her from sharing any information willingly.

I made it back to the house before Mom did. Such a relief. I also came to the disconcerting realization that her attention span and memory were waning. It was somewhat easy to distract her and gently fib about certain things, but her paranoia would perk up again unexpectedly and she would become wildly suspicious about everything. I was playing a behavioral guessing game at best.

November 2021

I turned the corner into the foyer and discovered a flat rate express mail envelope on the floor. I asked Mom about it. She grabbed it, clutched it to her chest, and informed me she had changed her legal documents again!

I asked if I could see the documents. She said I could review them after she had a chance to look them over. I didn't want to upset her, so I let it go. Later that day I found the envelope in her office and stashed it under a mattress. When she asked me what had happened to it, I told her she must have misplaced it. I was getting better at fibbing with finesse to protect her from herself and avoid more arguments.

Mom continued to change who held "the power" in her will, depending on her mood and which daughter was in favor that month. She alternated between giving me or my sister control over her assets with Nancy usually slated in the back-up role unless Mom got angry at her for some random reason. Thankfully, Nancy was consistently named as the point person for all medical matters.

I had another meeting with the elder law attorney and shared the revised documents with him. He agreed to contact Mom's attorney with a cease and desist letter to prevent more changes and charges. The most recent request to reshuffle had not been signed and notarized, so Nancy and I remained in control of Mom's health and finances.

I was always torn between digging too deeply and not deeply enough. During my monthly visits to LA, I hesitated when it came to taking a copy of the taxes or certain documents for fear Mom would discover my snooping. Each time, after I left her house, though, I would regret that I had not taken more as we tried to piece together a plan. We wanted to help her maintain a sense of control and prepare a plan with her cooperation and without extensive drama. Wishful thinking.

I took several pictures of her computer password cheat sheet to help us check account balances for overdrafts and duplicate payments. Some of Mom's passwords followed a standard pattern, but others were changed, crossed out, and, with random success, changed again to complicated strings of characters. Mom was paranoid and manic about maintaining control, which only made it more difficult for her to keep track of everything and just as difficult for us to help her.

Sometimes she would trust her grandsons to help, so we all worked together to distract her and share information. Our goal: to prevent her from locking us out of everything. Mom was highly suspicious of her family members but had no qualms about sharing her private financial information with random customer service reps eager to listen to her trials and tribulations.

Our Story: Finances

We had all been brought up with the value of living within your means. Saving was encouraged. Mom had always taken great pride in managing her finances, her business, and her investments wisely and responsibly. And she had always been organized and particular about paying bills in full and on time.

Yet she was desperately trying to keep paying basic bills. We should have been more aware of her shift from confidence to secrecy when it came to her bills. She was trying to conceal the fact that she was having trouble. She kept multiple notebooks and registers and cross-checked her statements multiple times, almost obsessively. She used check marks and highlighters to reconcile statements and then liquid paper to correct mistakes and start all over again.

She also began to accumulate notes of all kinds in the kitchen and her office area—notes on printouts, napkins, flyers, and envelopes, notes reminding her to follow up on a bill or call a vendor.

As the situation worsened, she spent considerable time on the phone badgering customer service reps and escalating her complaints to the highest level. She was convinced she was targeted for elder abuse fraud. This was partially true. She was clearly vulnerable. Mom had always been vocal about injustice so her behavior fit the bill perfectly. Maybe protesting gave her a sense of control she was used to having. It also allowed her to speak to a human being and assuage her loneliness.

Mom also had multiple versions of her password sheet listing dozens of accounts and websites. She primarily used one credit card, a debit card, and paid a few monthly bills for cable and utilities via check. She had set up a couple of bills for auto pay from her credit card, which became a huge nightmare after a simple, rare evening out with a girlfriend.

Mom perpetuated the pandemic by refusing to go anywhere or see anyone once the restrictions in Los Angeles County lifted. She was fully vaccinated and boosted but still made excuses about going out. The grocery store was the only place she felt safe and it served a purpose, mainly to restock her cigarettes!

Finally, she agreed to spend an evening at Disney Hall, a favorite outing, with her dear friend. They had held season tickets for several years. The night was a great success. She had a good time. A few weeks later, though, she complained about a fraudulent thirty-five-dollar charge on her credit card. She was determined to get it expunged. I noted the date and explained that it must have been a glass of wine for her and her friend at intermission during their night at Disney Hall. Sure enough, that's what it was, but she didn't remember the charge and continued to consider it fraudulent.

She began challenging other charges, canceling her card, and requesting replacement cards. She received five new cards within as many weeks, which messed up her auto payments and created a financial mess—mild problems by many standards, but a hassle all the same.

We finally utilized the legal power of attorney she had given Nancy to take control of all Mom's accounts. It took some time, as every institution had a slightly different process, but the effort was critical in protecting Mom's finances.

II. Prepare

HAVE THE CONVERSATION

FACT:
Two-thirds of adults don't have an advance directive.[33]

We need to normalize conversations about dementia. It is no different than being diagnosed with any physical disease. People used to whisper the "C word" for cancer because it wasn't talked about openly or publicly. Dementia is currently in that hush-hush category: the "D word" has become the new "C word" and that needs to change.

When there's a cancer diagnosis, neighborhoods set up meal trains and family members provide updates with regular blog posts. We need the same type of attention devoted to dementia, giving people the opportunity to rally around a person with dementia, their primary caregiver, and the family.

Death is inevitable for all of us. Yet most of us ignore it. Communication of any kind is difficult for humankind but we have to start somewhere. If you don't have a clue, you can begin with the *Death Over Dinner* or *Five Wishes* websites. The first suggests a formula, the culmination of expert advice, to host a "test dinner," a kind of rehearsal before gathering friends and family to have an empowering conversation about end-of-life planning. The second offers families an advance directive kit to aid them in such planning and make it a group experience.

33 www.americanbar.org/groups/law_aging/publications/bifocal/vol_37/issue_1_october2015/myths_and_facts_advance_directives/

Approaching the subject gently and gradually is important. Stressful holiday gatherings or rushed encounters probably are not the best time to bring up highly sensitive issues. Consult siblings, close friends, or other relatives who are concerned about the best approach. Family dynamics are complicated in the best of times and likely will become outrageously contentious if everyone is forced to face tough decisions in crisis mode. Whether you're ready or not, the crisis call will come eventually.

If you think about it, a couple typically spends eighteen months planning a wedding and nine months preparing for the arrival of a baby—both major life events. When that crisis call comes, a family member, then a newly crowned caregiver, may have twenty-four minutes to twenty-four hours to figure out how to manage the situation and make a plan pronto.

The stove is left on and a kitchen fire erupts; someone has a heart attack, a stroke, or a fall; there's been a car accident or unexpected incident. They all happen. Having a plan in place is critical. Start with legal/financial matters or begin by creating a healthcare directive. Wherever you start, the important thing is to open the conversation. Every family situation is different. Find the easiest starting point for you and yours.

If you suspect your parent has mild cognitive impairment or dementia, it behooves you to get things moving sooner versus later. Laws vary considerably by state and tax implications play a part, too. Start with the basics and enlist help from professionals even if it seems expensive. If a plan or document is prepared improperly, the cost will be higher in the long run. Educate yourself on the basics first. There are countless free webinars and resources to get you started, including an AARP article entitled, "How to Stop Stalling On Getting a Will and Estate Plan."[34]

---

34 www.aarp.org/retirement/planning-for-retirement/info-2020/how-to-write-wills-estate-plans.html

CONVERSATION STARTERS

Five Wishes
www.fivewishes.org:

> The nation's only advanced care planning program, which features an easy-to-use workbook that becomes a legal advance directive.

Death Over Dinner
deathoverdinner.org:

> An interactive adventure that transforms the often-dreaded conversation into an empowering experience.

The Conversation Project
theconversationproject.org:

> An initiative to help everyone talk about their wishes for care through the end of life.

LEGAL DOCUMENTS

It is imperative to locate and take inventory of legal documents: will, trust, power of attorney, living will, and healthcare directive, to name a few. Each state has different rules regarding estate planning, how assets get distributed, and whether an inheritance tax is assessed. A trust can be helpful in some states but not necessary in others. Financial assets can be transferred to family members outside a will via beneficiary designation forms. These terms and documents are complicated and confusing. Take the time to become familiar with some of the basics and ask questions of professionals. Each state is very different. Having assets in multiple states changes the dynamic, too.

When preparing documents, consider three imperative factors—what assets you have, who will receive those assets, and who will distribute those assets, namely, an executor. Basic forms for many documents are available online. Some estates are less complicated than others. Remember, you get what you pay for, so focus on the basics first and use referrals to shop around for professionals you can trust.

FINANCIAL POWER OF ATTORNEY (POA)

The two most pressing and important documents to draft sooner versus later are the financial power of attorney and the medical power of attorney. The latter is sometimes called a healthcare directive. Probate laws vary by state. Forms and terminology vary as well.

A financial power of attorney document can be specific or extensive in the authority it grants. The form can limit power to financial transactions or extend to cover legal and tax matters. If a person or parent designates someone as having power of attorney over their assets, they are still able to spend and donate their own money. The POA does not revoke their control over their own assets; it enables the designated POA to act on their behalf.

The person creating the legal documents and giving power to another trusted individual is called the grantor. The person the grantor trusts to act on the grantor's behalf is called the agent.

There are five types of power of attorney: durable, springing, general, limited, and digital:

1. **A durable power of attorney**, typically used in estate planning, is effective immediately upon signature. In most states, a court will presume a POA is durable.[35]

   With a non-durable power of attorney, the agent's power to act on the grantor's behalf stops if the grantor becomes incapacitated or dies. This type of document is usually employed for limited periods of time or for specific purposes involving signing documents or approving payments.

2. **A springing power of attorney** also has strings attached. It requires some condition to be met before it "springs" into action. Commonly, a springing power of attorney requires a physician to declare the grantor incapacitated, and unable to make their own decisions, before the agent can act on the grantor's behalf. For instance, the grantor may be in a coma.

---

35 www.freewill.com/learn/5-types-of-power-of-attorney

3. While **a general power of attorney** gives an agent a fair amount of power over the grantor's affairs, it doesn't offer carte blanche. Many times, for instance, an agent can't make a will on behalf of a grantor.

   a. A grantor can offer a limited financial POA to an agent for particular asset related tasks, such as paying bills, doing banking, filing taxes, or selling a piece of real estate.

   b. In this age of the Internet, most of us have a significant digital footprint, including random photos and important information stored somewhere in the cloud. It is prudent to consider designating someone to manage your devices, accounts, and passwords.[36] Talk to your attorney about adding a digital designee to your power of attorney document.

One or another of these types and considerations probably applies to your situation.

MEDICAL POWER OF ATTORNEY

In a medical power of attorney document, also called a healthcare power of attorney, you appoint a healthcare agent, or proxy, to act on your behalf in medical matters, including surgeries, treatments, and even which practitioners and institutions are used to administer care. If you make this document durable, your proxy is empowered to keep acting on your behalf even if you cannot communicate your desires because of a degenerative condition such as dementia or stroke or because you are under anesthesia.[37]

A second part of medical planning includes a living will, which stipulates what extraordinary measures you do or do not want taken to save your life, including resuscitation, feeding tubes, and certain medications. A living will also records your preferences for other decisions, such as organ donation and pain management.

---

36 www.amazon.com/55-Essential-Legal-Documents-Need/dp/1610352580
37 www.freewill.com/learn/5-types-of-power-of-attorney

Both documents are considered "healthcare advance directives." While you can prepare your own advance directives, they will only be valid if you follow legal protocols.[38]

In some states they can be one document but in others, they are two separate documents. Each state has its own forms.[39]

GUARDIANSHIP OR CONSERVATORSHIP

Some seniors do not have family members living, willing, or able to participate as caregivers or guardians. In those instances the state court can appoint an individual to step into this role. Again, terminology varies by state. Some states use the term "guardianship," others "conservatorship." A guardianship can be established for an estate, a person, or both. A guardian is appointed when a person is deemed unable to make decisions for themselves. Guardians are fiduciaries who must follow significantly detailed protocols and reporting requirements. The role holds a high degree of responsibility and should not be taken lightly. Any suspected abuse or mismanagement of funds should be reported to Adult Protective Services.[40]

Similarly, if your parent refuses to move or refuses help of any kind, you may need to enlist the help of an elder law attorney and consider guardianship or conservatorship. Since the process is long and expensive, the Family Caregiver Alliance advises giving the matter careful consideration before undertaking it.[41]

LAST WILLS AND TESTAMENTS

In a common "I Love You"/Sweetheart Will, each spouse leaves their whole estate to the other and then, many times, to their children to split. Each spouse prepares a will that mirrors the other. Even if property is owned jointly, each individual needs to make their own will.[42]

---

38 www.americanbar.org/groups/law_aging/publications/bifocal/vol_37/issue_1_october2015/myths_and_facts_advance_directives/
39 www.caringinfo.org/planning/advance-directives/by-state/
40 www.hhs.gov/answers/programs-for-families-and-children/how-do-i-report-elder-abuse/index.html
41 www.caregiver.org/resource/conservatorship-and-guardianship
42 www.legalzoom.com/articles/the-basics-of-i-love-you-wills

TRUSTS: IRREVOCABLE, REVOCABLE, QTIP

Laws governing trusts vary by state. In some they are useful in protecting assets while in others, they are unnecessary. Evaluate the estate planning situation in your state before setting up a trust.

A financial trust will control how your assets are distributed and managed after your death and are beneficial in several ways. They allow you to choose beneficiaries for particular assets, identify the rules and timetables for distributions, avoid probate, reduce tax liability, protect vulnerable family members, and keep your assets private, unlike a last will and testament, which is filed with the government and becomes a public document.

A trust also allows you to establish a plan for your own long-term care and have your trustee manage your assets in the event you cannot act on your own behalf.

In setting up a trust, you first must decide how much control you want over your trust assets. Then you'll know whether you want an irrevocable or revocable trust. There are important differences between them.

An irrevocable trust cannot be changed once it is created, not even by the person who established it, the grantor. Such a trust can only be changed or revoked by court order or under limited, strictly defined circumstances.

On the other hand, you can change, or even revoke, a revocable trust while you're still alive. Once you die, however, the trust cannot be changed and becomes irrevocable.

The duties of a named executor in a last will and testament are different than those of a trustee. The former executes the directions set forth in your will but a trustee gets rights to actually hold assets on your behalf.[43]

Another type of trust—a qualified terminable interest property (QTIP) trust—provides income to a surviving spouse and holds the balance of the estate in trust. Once that spouse dies, the remainder of the trust is paid to beneficiaries as the grantor stipulated. A QTIP trust is particularly, but not exclusively, useful when a grantor wants to provide for a current spouse and has beneficiaries from a previous marriage.[44]

---

43 njelc.com/why-you-should-create-a-last-will-and-testament-and-a-trust/
44 www.investopedia.com/terms/q/qtip.asp

ELDER LAW ATTORNEYS

Even if you already have a will and your legal affairs in order, it may be wise to enlist the help of an attorney who specializes in elder law. They are familiar with estate planning and know how you can best manage benefits, care, and placement options for your loved one.

While estate planning is different from elder law, the two overlap. Before you choose a lawyer, understand their area of specialty. Do not hesitate to ask questions about how to protect your family's assets so you can afford to get your parent the best care.

Finding appropriately qualified attorneys is easy when you know where to look. Here are a few organizations and an online locator that can help:

4. **The National Academy of Elder Law Attorneys** (NAELA),[45] a nonprofit association whose mission, per its website, is to "educate, inspire, serve, and provide community to attorneys with practices in elder and special needs law." Its members are across the US and in Canada, Australia, and the UK.

5. **The National Elder Law Foundation** (NELF),[46] the only national organization that certifies practitioners of elder and special needs law. The American Bar Association certifies NELF's Certified Elder Law Attorney (CELA) designation.

6. **National Association of Estate Planners & Councils** (NAEPC),[47] an organization that recognizes, supports, and educates those who hold Estate Planning Law Specialist (EPLS) certification.

7. **Elder Care Locator**,[48] a clearinghouse of resources for all things elderly, searchable by zip code.

---

45 naela.org/
46 nelf.org/
47 www.naepc.org/
48 eldercare.acl.gov/Public/Index.aspx

FINANCIAL DOCUMENTS

Seniors primarily worry about not being a burden to their children and wanting to leave a little bit of money to them. Taking inventory of their financial situation and having the correct forms and documents in place can help alleviate those concerns. Many people shy away from talking about personal wealth. Ignoring the topic now, though, will only make things worse later. Do you want your assets going to family members you choose or locked up in probate where the attorneys will profit? What do you do? Have the conversation!

BENEFICIARY DESIGNATIONS

You can transfer assets, such as portfolios, insurance policies, and IRA payouts directly to family members by designating them as your beneficiary. When beneficiary forms are in place, they take precedence over a will. Certificates of Deposit (CDs) require a Payable on Death form on file or the asset goes through probate. Each asset and institution has unique forms to designate a beneficiary. You can name an individual or an entity, such as a trust or nonprofit, or you can name your estate as the beneficiary of a financial or retirement account when it is opened or a life insurance policy when it is established.

When a major life change, such as a birth, marriage, or divorce, occurs, an account holder should revisit their accounts and update their beneficiaries.

A beneficiary will receive the remaining balance in your account or the death benefit from your policy when you die. If your primary beneficiary predeceases you, the asset or benefit goes to your contingent beneficiary. If your estate is your beneficiary, your financial team will turn to your will for directions on how to distribute your money and to whom.[49]

BANK ACCOUNT COSIGNERS VERSUS CO-OWNERS

Authorized signers typically can make deposits and withdrawals, including writing checks and using the account's debit card. They can only act on behalf of the account owner and have no personal ownership rights to the assets. Having financial power of attorney for someone also may allow you to access and manage their bank account.

As co-owners, both parties are able to access and withdraw funds without the other's permission. Each can also talk to the bank about the account without the consent of the other. A co-owner is different than a joint owner: while a co-owner can act on behalf of the owner to access the account, they are not responsible for fees and don't claim the account as an asset. Each bank or financial institution may have different terminology or rules regarding co-ownership. Clarify before making changes or adding individuals.

WEALTH ADVISORS

It is a good idea to take inventory of your parent's current assets so you know exactly how much money is available and can plan appropriately for their needs and care. Also ask where they keep important documents and papers. Consult with a wealth advisor or certified financial planner (CFP), which is different from a certified public accountant (CPA).[50] They can, however, work together for tax strategy investment planning.

Financial planning certification is the standard of excellence in financial planning.[51]

CERTIFIED PUBLIC ACCOUNTANTS

Some people do their taxes with simple software programs but, as the old adage goes, you get what you pay for. Enlisting a

---

49 trustandwill.com/learn/beneficiary-designation
50 www.aicpa-cima.com/home
51 www.cfp.net/

professional to prepare tax documents can help with deductions. They can examine past returns and assess asset management to accurately calculate tax liability, which helps you plan for your parent's future.

HOW TO PAY FOR IT ALL

If you are dirt poor or filthy rich, you have access to programs or resources to cover care for your loved one. If you're in the "forgotten middle," however, you will struggle through the system and may wind up "spending down" your parent's assets so they can qualify for Medicaid. While those who can afford private pay can place their loved one in a "cruise ship" version of senior living communities, they still endure the stress and guilt that come with putting mom or dad in a foreign place. And they still have to navigate the medical, financial, and legal decisions that need to be made as well as all the crises that come with the territory.

As I mentioned what I was going through with my mom in passing conversations, I was shocked to learn just how many people were in the same situation. I tend to be effusive about everything happening in my life and eagerly soaked up the stories people shared with me. There were some common themes and threads, but just as every birth story is unique, each aging parent story is ripe with unpredictability we could all relate to and learn from.

One scenario is the adult child who is acutely aware that one parent is failing but cannot intervene because the other parent insists on caring for their spouse and refuses to leave the home. Children have a difficult time overcoming an ingrained sense of obedience. And they can only do so much when a parent makes an unwise decision. A devoted spouse may mean well but end up compromising their own health. Then the adult child is faced with two chronically ill parents, adding anguish to the equation and putting added strain on finances.

Have the conversation and get the power of attorney for finances and healthcare done sooner rather than later. Not an easy endeavor, I know, but necessary.

Even with all the apps and connectivity and the saturation of social media today, I have found that the people who are most successful in managing a tough care situation usually find their caregivers through good old-fashioned word of mouth. Hopefully, the shame and stigma around dementia is dissipating so people are more open to discussing it. I suggest reaching out where you feel most comfortable and having faith the right solution will present itself after some investigation.

A combination of Facebook groups, local and virtual support groups, neighbors, parishioners, and coworkers make for a good starting strategy. You will quickly discover that you are not alone in this endeavor. If you are not comfortable sharing your personal situation with others, geriatric care managers and certified senior advisors in the business of eldercare and placement can help.

Each state and situation comes with its own challenges and rules, including filial responsibility laws that in some cases could require adult children to financially provide for the care of their elderly parents.[52] So you will have to dig and have lots of discussions to find the right solutions for your family. Having the difficult conversations and practicing a little due diligence pays off. If you wait until you're in crisis mode to seek solutions, you'll make mistakes.

---

52 www.caregiverrelief.com/filial-responsibility-laws/

RESOURCES FOR FINANCIAL SOLUTIONS

Here are some ways to evaluate the cost of your parent's care and resources to get help:

Elder Care Solutions
www.eldercaresolutionsinc.com/for-those-aging-and-caring:

> Organization that provides affordable guidance sessions and cost analysis tools to help individuals and families assess the high cost of care.

**Pharmaceutical Aid for the Aged
and Disabled (PAAD) and Senior Gold**
www.payingforseniorcare.com/new-jersey/senior-gold-paad:

> Drug assistance programs that offer low-cost medications, and even free drug plans, to New Jersey residents age sixty-five and older and those with disabilities

**Veterans Affairs (VA) Aid and Attendance
and Household Allowance**
www.va.gov/pension/aid-attendance-housebound:

> Monthly payments that supplement a monthly VA pension for qualifying veterans and survivors.

BOOKS

I read extensively to learn as much as I could about dementia and senior care. Here are a few of my favorite books.[53]

The 36-Hour Day: A Family Guide to Caring for People Who Have Alzheimer Disease and Other Dementias
by Nancy L. Mace and Peter V. Rabins

***The Dutiful Daughter's Guide to Caregiving:
A Practical Memoir***
by Judith Henry

---

53 I also review books on Instagram. Visit @dementiabookreview

Elderhood: Redefining Aging, Transforming Medicine, Reimagining Life
by Louise Aronson

How to Care for Aging Parents: A One-Stop Resource for All Your Medical, Financial, Housing, and Emotional Issues
by Virginia Morris

Keeper: One House, Three Generations, and a Journey into Alzheimer's
by Andrea Gillies

Learning to Speak Alzheimer's: A Groundbreaking Approach for Everyone Dealing with the Disease
by Joanne Koenig Coste

Life: The Next Phase
by Mary Beth Cozza, Helen B. Hempel, and Jodi Hempel

Passages in Caregiving: Turning Chaos into Confidence
by Gail Sheehy

CRITICAL CONTACTS FOLDER

Being organized is crucial as you navigate every twist and turn in your parent's world. You'll be called upon to produce all kinds of records, cards, and information on demand. You need to develop a system of storing all critical documents so they are readily available.

I took photos of Mom's driver's license and Social Security, Medicare, and insurance cards, and stored them in Favorites on my phone for easy access. I also use a combination of three-ring binders and color-coded folders to manage her documents—green for financial statements and bills, blue for medical documents, and red for legal documents.

The important thing is to create a simple system that makes sense to you. Here is a checklist of documents to secure and organize:

- ☐ Password list for all online accounts, including email, portals, credit card accounts, utilities, bank and mortgage accounts, etc.
- ☐ Bank statements
- ☐ Birth certificate
- ☐ Clergy (priest/imam/rabbi/spiritual advisor)
- ☐ Credit card statements
- ☐ Death certificate (spouse)

- ☐ Dentist
- ☐ Doctors (optometrist/ophthalmologist/retina specialist)
- ☐ Doctors (primary care)
- ☐ Doctor specialists (cardiologist, dermatologist, geriatrician, gynecologist, internist, orthopedist, podiatrist, rheumatologist, urologist)
- ☐ Driver's license
- ☐ Faith community members (name/address/phone/email)
- ☐ Family members (name/address/phone/email)
- ☐ Financial advisor/investment statements
- ☐ Friends (name/address/phone/email)
- ☐ House records, including maintenance, repair, and improvement projects
- ☐ Insurance policies and contacts, including house, car, health, etc.
- ☐ IRA, retirement, pension statements
- ☐ Legal documents, including trust, will, powers of attorney, healthcare directive
- ☐ Marriage certificate
- ☐ Medicare card
- ☐ Medicare supplemental policy card
- ☐ Military discharge papers
- ☐ Mortgage statements
- ☐ Neighbors (name/address/phone/email)
- ☐ Passport
- ☐ Phone bill statements
- ☐ Physical therapist

- ☐ Psychiatrist/psychologist/licensed clinical social worker/counselor
- ☐ Social Security card
- ☐ Tax records and accountant contact information
- ☐ Vehicle title of ownership
- ☐ Veterinarian/kennel for pets
- ☐ Water/electric/pest control records

Our Story: Social Security

The Social Security Administration is a critical contact for everyone. Mom's monthly checks continued to be deposited in her bank account, which Nancy managed as power of attorney. I had Mom's online *My Social Security* account ID and password, but it required more verification through email and phone codes, so I chose the snail mail option to receive communications from the agency. I knew any mail eventually would be forwarded to Nancy's house. She and I had initiated United States Post Office (USPS) mail forwarding, available as a courtesy service for one year, when we cleaned out Mom's house for sale in January 2022. The USPS will extend the forwarding period for a fee.

A Social Security Administration letter arrived in early September with instructions on how to change the way we received codes for Mom's online account. It contained a one-time reset code with instructions and an expiration date. We were busy, then Nancy took a trip to Europe. When she returned, we focused on this issue before the code deadline expired.

The process worked—up until the point when a legalese waiver popped up on our screen with a bunch of warnings about anyone other than Mom using this account. I wasn't prepared to sign that and figured there must be another way since dementia is not a unique problem. I thought they just might have a form or process for people in our situation.

October 20, 2022

I called the national 800-772-1213 Social Security number and waited on hold for forty minutes to speak to a human. Hannah asked me for standard information and then for a bank account routing number, which I did not have handy. I asked for patience while I rifled through the fifteen folders I'd created for my mother's documents. She waited for maybe a minute and told me she could not wait any longer for me to find them. I told her I waited forty minutes to get a human and she should cut me some slack. At that point she got combative and demanded my information since I was clearly a scammer trying to cheat my mother out of her money.

I demanded Hannah's last name, agent number, and location, which she would not disclose. After all, she had the luxury of complete anonymity and zero accountability.

After we both calmed down, I asked Hannah what the standard procedure might be for a parent suffering from dementia. She told me I needed to request to become a "representative payee" and that I should make an appointment at the nearest Social Security office to begin the process. I explained I had already been in the 800 number loop and the website gave the standard national 800 number for every Social Security office location. So how could I call the local office to make an appointment?

She gave me the local office number and said I would need to give the local agent my own proof of identification and, to verify my mother's dementia diagnosis, the name and phone number of my mother's doctor.

October 21, 2022

I called the local New Jersey office number and was told they do not make appointments at all, for anything. (Thanks, Hannah.) I had to go in person, take a number, and wait to talk to a human. I asked if the office was usually filled with visitors. The man who answered the phone replied that he worked in a back office and had no idea about the volume of people in the waiting room. I took a book with me and prepared to wait and get it done.

When I arrived "MUST WEAR FACE MASK" signs were plastered all over the walls and doors. I entered the office and approached the buff and tough security guard who dwarfed the desk he was sitting at. He wore his face mask as a chin strap. I had missed the sign instructing me to use the kiosk to sign in, and he politely redirected me.

After several failed attempts to use the touch screen, he bellowed instructions as if he had repeated them hundreds of times before.

"Just tap the screen," he said. "Don't hold your finger. Go to the center ... On the line. No, higher up ... " *Oh my God!* I witnessed this same instruction scenario play out several more times as I patiently waited my turn to speak to a human.

The tough and buff but polite security guard instructed everyone in the waiting area that *all* chimes, beeps, ringers, email notifications, and social media sounds on their phones should be turned off for the duration of our wait. No phone conversations were allowed in the waiting room. Inevitably, a forbidden ping or song or ringtone would break the stifled silence, causing the guard to roll his eyes and repeat his mantra.

One poor guy couldn't get his video sound feed to stop and offered his sincerest apologies. A woman asked if she was allowed to use the wall outlet to charge her phone. Yes, she could.

Thankfully, my number was called soon. My wait in the chime-free room was significantly shorter than my Muzak-drone time on the phone the previous day. I took my binders and letters down the hallway to window No. 9 where the agent was, thankfully, familiar with the concept of a "representative payee." When I reached for the physician letters, though, he stopped me.

"You need to have a phone interview for that process," he informed me. "The first available interview time is in eight weeks."

I asked what documents and/or information I would be required to have on hand for that interview. He had no idea. I was to just sit by the phone on the date/time instructed and wait for that agent to tell me—something.

Eight weeks later I was pleasantly surprised when the call came in on schedule. I discussed the details with the agent, who was attentive and informative. Ultimately, we decided it was not necessary for me to become a representative payee. At that juncture our best course of action was to continue to have Mom's Social Security check deposited into her checking account, which Nancy actively managed as her financial power of attorney. This plan would suffice temporarily. The policy specifically says:

> Family members often use a power of attorney as another way to handle a family member's finances. For our purposes, a power of attorney isn't an acceptable way to manage a person's monthly benefits. We recognize only a designated representative payee for handling the beneficiary's funds.[54]

The initial purpose of this process was to make sure any mail from Social Security reached us after the USPS mail forwarding period expired. I am not sure but I believe that when I chatted with the man at window No. 9, he changed my address and Mom's address in the system while we met, fulfilling my purpose. I provided our Social Security numbers. He updated everything. My address on file was twenty years old, probably because that was about the time I left the workforce to stay home and raise my kids. I hadn't earned wages since then.

I learned that even though Mom's Social Security money was being deposited and carefully managed by Nancy, my not registering as a representative payee could still have repercussions: we would be powerless to correct any situation that might arise if there was a clerical error or fraudulent claim against Mom's account. Sometimes credit card or insurance companies will agree to talk to a child, spouse, or agent if the account holder gives verbal agreement over the phone in a conference call. This is not the case with Social Security, which is strict about following procedures and will not allow a person with dementia to express opinions and make decisions on a call.

---

54 www.ssa.gov/pubs/EN-05-10076.pdf

As my reality game of whack-a-mole continued, I kicked the can down the road on this issue to resolve at a later date. My family finally relocated to Arizona in July 2023. We planned to move Mom to a memory care unit in Arizona within six months. I revisited this issue with a trip to my local Arizona Social Security office to once again investigate becoming a representative payee for Mom.

To get you started on the right foot, know that the Social Security Administration has *A Guide for Representative Payees*[55] and that, while an adult child representative payee still must file an annual accounting of how they spent their parent's Social Security benefit, other payees, as of June 13, 2022, do not.[56]

Note that the Social Security Administration will assign a representative payee—an individual or organization—for recipients who don't have someone willing or able to fill the role.[57]

---

[55] www.ssa.gov/pubs/EN-05-10076.pdf
[56] www.federalregister.gov/documents/2022/06/13/2022-12682/reducing-burden-on-families-acting-as-representative-payees-of-social-security-payments
[57] www.ssa.gov/payee/

MEDICAL MATTERS

The entire healthcare system is designed to treat and cure, not to let go. What do you need to do? Have the conversation! Make sure your loved one gets to put on paper, in advance, the healthcare choices they prefer when times get tough. It's best if they make these decisions while they're calm and can articulate their wishes.

"The discussion should consider the possible, probable, and problematic scenarios," says Chris Kellogg of Nightingale New Jersey Eldercare Navigators, who shared his expertise on the *Happy to Help* radio show. "Erratic emotion overrides common sense in a crisis situation. Discussing and documenting these decisions in a calm, intentional setting is preferred."

Helpful hint: Phrase your concerns using the word "I" when talking with your parent or loved one instead of itemizing all the things they have done "wrong" to create cause for concern. Choose your words carefully to address this sensitive subject. Start with "I'm concerned because—"

Designating a healthcare proxy and drafting a medical power of attorney document is not an end in itself. This document leads to even more documents. It begins a journey. Keep in mind that medical decisions become more specific as a patient's health deteriorates.

Let's take a look at other documents and matters a healthcare proxy person should tend to.

DO NOT RESUSCITATE

A Do Not Resuscitate (DNR) is a single medical order that instructs a healthcare team not to perform cardiopulmonary resuscitation (CPR) on a patient if their breathing or blood flow stops. It is written by a doctor after speaking with the patient. If the patient is not conscious or able to communicate, the doctor will consult the patient's proxy or family.[58]

POLST

The Physician Orders for Life-Sustaining Treatment (POLST) is a form designed for seriously ill or frail people. It is a set of medical orders that allows patients to accept or decline a variety of potentially lifesaving medical interventions, including CPR, airway management, and artificially administered fluids and nutrition. This document must be signed by a physician. The official document sometimes goes by different names, such as Medical Orders for Life-Sustaining Treatment (MOLST), Medical Orders for Scope of Treatment (MOST), or Physician Orders for Scope of Treatment (POST). Since it is usually printed on colored paper, the document is sometimes referenced as "the pink form" or "the green form."

A POLST form is portable, meaning it will be honored across all treatment settings, not just in a hospital. POLST programs are run by states.[59]

A designated healthcare proxy person should have a copy of all relevant documents, which should be kept within reach, not locked away. Some people store them in their overnight suitcases or tape them to the refrigerator or bedroom door.

---

58 medlineplus.gov/ency/patientinstructions/000473.htm
59 polst.org/state-polst-programs/

MEDICATIONS

Scientists do not definitively know what causes dementia. Consequently, there is no way to predict who will develop dementia and who will not. And there is no cure. The potential for profit in this area is astronomical. Be wary of any programs, pills, books, banter, or claims from savvy scammers who prey on hope and promise something too good to be true.

Common sense would suggest that what is good for the body is good for the brain. Diet, exercise, sleep, socialization, and purpose roughly round out the top five. You can't cram all that into a pill or a single program.

As of this writing, there are several FDA-approved medications for Alzheimer's and certain other types of dementia. They focus on easing symptoms and slowing the disease's progression. For instance, recent medical literature shows people in early-stage Alzheimer's may benefit from lecanemab.[60] Anyone considering medication should consult their physician in order to understand the potential benefits and be aware of possible side effects.

One of the most commonly prescribed drugs for mild to moderate Alzheimer's disease is donepezil (Aricept), a cholinesterase inhibitor that prevents the breakdown of acetylcholine in the brain. This chemical, key in memory-making, thinking, and reasoning, is present in lower levels in the brains of Alzheimer's patients. Aricept will slow, not stop, the disease.[61] Other cholinesterase inhibitors sometimes prescribed

---

60 www.alz.org/news/2022/statement-lecanemab-phase-three-full-results
61 www.drugs.com/aricept.html

for mild to moderate Alzheimer's are galantamine (Razadyne) and rivastigmine (Exelon).[62]

In moderate to severe cases, donepezil is sometimes combined with memantine (Namenda); the latter regulates glutamate, a chemical that helps the brain process information.[63]

Risperidone (Risperdal), used to treat schizophrenia, also changes chemicals in the brain but bears a FDA "black box warning" that identifies its serious, even life-threatening, side effects: it increases the risk of "cerebrovascular adverse events" and even death for older adults with dementia-related psychosis.[64]

Our Story: Medications

Shortly after mom moved into the senior residence, Nancy met with the medical professional staff members to review Mom's meds and reassess her needs. We knew what prescription meds she had been taking (or failing to take) in California. She was also given various meds while in an emergency room and at a psych facility in New Jersey. (More on both later.)

Nancy and I were present for Mom's initial meeting with the nurse practitioner. Mom was pleased to have an audience of three. Knowing we were there to discuss her meds, she wanted to make her views clear. She prepared to record everything we discussed in a notebook.

Mom took control and began by emphatically declaring her desire to die. She had lived a full life, she said, and did not appreciate being placed in this facility against her will.

"It's my time to go," she added, matter-of-factly. "I'm ready."

The nurse practitioner politely explained to Mom that physician-assisted suicide is legal in some states but not in Maryland. Nancy and I proclaimed that we loved Mom but were not prepared to go to jail to grant her wish to die.

---

62 www.alz.org/alzheimers-dementia/treatments/medications-for-memory
63 www.webmd.com/drugs/2/drug-77936/namenda-oral/details
64 www.ncbi.nlm.nih.gov/pmc/articles/PMC7256877/

Patiently, the nurse practitioner repeated phrases and spelled out drug names so Mom could write them down. We all discussed dosages and frequency. The memory care staff would bring Mom her meds. She was no longer responsible for managing them but she wanted to be aware of them.

"What about this Risperidone script?" the nurse practitioner asked Nancy. "It's a black box drug."

"What's a black box drug?" I asked.

"A drug gets that designation when it can cause severe side effects or imminent death," she replied. Mom had just given an earnest speech about her desire to die.

"Perfect!" I said, jokingly.

The psych hospital had started Mom on this drug. The nurse practitioner took her off it.

FAMILY DYNAMICS

Family drama is everywhere and only intensifies when health, wealth, and literal life and death decisions come into play. When things get serious, childhood grievances can resurface or sprout anew. Once again, know you are not alone in dealing with a fierce family dynamic.

Communication is critical and best started earlier rather than later to avoid emotional turmoil. Easier said than done. Preparing early is important. Build a plan of care that caters to the strengths of each child or relative. For instance, some siblings are willing to take on the heavy lifting of daily caregiving if someone else handles the legal and financial footwork.

Since people have different perspectives and opinions on every aspect of care, the blame game can escalate quickly. Gaslighting and contact blocking are quite common, but you can control who you call to vent, ask for advice, or enlist for assistance. We will help you build your self-care and support network in the next section.

Hopefully, you can be proactive and start gathering resources and enlisting help from family members, friends, and professionals before an acute incident requires immediate action. Creating a plan ahead of time is better than making rash decisions under emotional distress but understand this: you won't necessarily be able to implement your plan on *your* timeline when other people, including your afflicted parent, are involved.

Caregiver Consultant Deb Hallisey discusses this potential disconnect in her book, *Your Caregiver Relationship Contract*: "If your loved one has the mental capacity, he or she has the right to make the wrong decision."[65] They still have final say-so on how they live their life, even if it makes yours more difficult!

Waiting to implement a plan can be the toughest part. Still, it behooves you to be prepared.

Our Story: Legal Musical Chairs

Mom had originally created a will, trust, and other documents in 2003, but they needed updating. Nancy had flown out to LA in fall 2019 to follow up on more doctor appointments and focus on reviewing Mom's legal documents. She wanted to ensure things were in order. While she was there, Nancy encouraged Mom to remove her from much of the responsibility for her affairs and bestow it to her daughters. Nancy is, after all, Mom's older sister. Mom obliged initially, but at some point she changed almost everything back to the way it was, once again making Nancy the primary caretaker of her assets.

To avoid swapping daughter names on legal documents each time she was annoyed with one of us, Mom felt it was easier to default everything to Nancy. This scenario often plays out in families.

Our Story: Same Play, Different Actors

We obtained a list of elder law attorneys from the hospital system. I was determined to find someone to help us work through this dementia dilemma. I spent an afternoon dialing down the list. If I reached an automated system that was too cumbersome, I moved on. If I sensed the office was too big or busy or self-absorbed, I kept dialing.

I wanted to find a female attorney if I could. My mother was always an advocate for women-owned businesses, and she ran

---

65 www.amazon.com/Your-Caregiver-Relationship-Contract-expectations-ebook/dp/B07WSH318K

one herself. A plethora of my peers are attorneys, so I figured I wouldn't have to look too hard to find a good one. After about a dozen phone calls and inquiries, I reached an actual human—a male elder law attorney who is slightly elder himself. I bonded with him immediately.

He answered the phone personally. His voice was genuine and relatable. He also reminded me of Bert, my late stepfather. I got the gut feel confirmation I was searching for. We talked for about an hour. He listened to my plight and we shared some personal stories.

Bob's father-in-law had suffered with dementia and, in his final years, lived in a facility a few blocks from Bob's office. That was the clincher. Bob understood the law, but he also understood the disease from personal experience. He knew what we were going through as a family but could be an objective voice of reason when we were mired in emotion.

I made plans to meet with Bob in person during my next trip to LA. COVID-19 had calmed down and he was comfortable with me coming to his office if I wore a mask. I am fine on the phone and proficient at Zoom, but I still prefer personal interaction when possible.

When I met with Bob, I shared the family dynamics and the predicament we found ourselves in. He listened attentively and kindly chuckled at the story. He had seen this movie before. Same play, different actors. He said that when older people need help, there is always someone with their hand out, someone who has checked out, and someone left dealing with all the logistics and dynamics. We fit the mold.

We had learned that, due to the Mom factor, our situation was more complicated. By nature she is stubborn, feisty, and defiant and so she refused to give up her freedom or her house. One cannot blame her. Many of the eldercare professionals we talked to admitted that Mom's situation was particularly challenging. She was lucid enough to wreak havoc on our efforts to keep her safe and protect her assets. Due to the diagnosis, her rational reasoning was no longer functioning, though. Mom believed only what she chose to believe.

She refused to believe, for instance, that she was running out of money and could no longer stay in her house. Yet her expenses were three times her monthly income. I did the math with her on paper and showed her financial statements. Reality still didn't sink in. Instead she insisted she magically made all of her money back in the market a month after she withdrew funds. It did not matter that her financial statements did not reflect her beliefs.

Mom had been a powerful, successful businesswoman who always paid her bills on time, invested wisely, and carefully monitored her finances. In her mind she was independently wealthy with the freedom and ability to do as she pleased—and she was not leaving her house.

We hoped Bob could help us figure out a way to coax her out of the house. We discussed establishing a conservatorship and what that would entail. The process was lengthy, costly, and messy, but it seemed like it could be our only option short of kidnapping her and forcefully removing her from the home!

Nancy and I continued discussing ways to get Mom to fly to the East Coast. We worked on several parallel plans at any given time but also stayed in touch with a couple of senior living facilities in the LA area. Mom clearly loved California and wanted to stay in the sunny state, but we wanted her on the East Coast where we could visit and monitor her health. We needed her close for convenience and peace of mind.

My sister lived in LA but had proven many times over that she was so busy, she couldn't help much with Mom.

Our research emphasized the importance of having family nearby to regularly visit residents in senior care facilities. It was good for the resident, of course, but also appeared to make a difference in how the staff treats the resident. It's good for staff to know that family members are stopping by frequently and paying close attention to how their loved one is being cared for.

Bob was a huge help in walking us through the legal procedures and implications of our choices. He also lent a personal touch that was critical to our mental well-being as we endured the uncertainty of it all.

Family dynamics are challenging enough on any given day.

One good crisis can throw an otherwise amicable relationship into chaos, especially when money is involved. Some relatives come out of the woodwork when they sense a change of health status that could indicate a windfall. I knew my brother would not come looking for a handout. He had checked out long ago: he and my mother had not spoken in nearly twenty years.

My brother and his wife live in Arkansas, many states away from wherever Mom would end up living. I respect their choice to remain distant. My brother would not participate in figuring out Mom's future, and I was fine with that.

Besides, Mom was not wealthy. We were moving her out of her home for safety and security reasons and to liquidate her primary asset to pay for her care. Senior living, especially memory care, is expensive.

My sister who lived near Mom in California helped her tour local senior living places. Nancy toured several places with Mom, too. Mom humored them both by playing along. She talked a good game but had no intention of going anywhere.

III. Build a Plan of Care

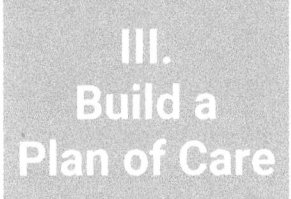

DON'T GO IT ALONE

FACT:
Thirty percent of caregivers pass away before the loved one they are caring for.[66]

Andrea Cohen, cofounder of the Boston-based HouseWorks, an in-home private care company, says most family caregivers don't look for solutions until a crisis hits.

It doesn't have to be that way if you build a plan of care for your loved one with inherent safeguards and contingencies. Convinced? Good, but know that the loved one you're caring for may not be ready to cooperate, which is their rightful prerogative. At first you may have to play a waiting game. If things go sideways before a plan is in place, you may find yourself scrambling—and that's just the way it is on what Cohen calls this "journey with no predictable end."

When I think of my father's reluctance to make a care plan, I'm reminded of the stubborn old coot story in Atul Gawande's bestseller, *Being Mortal.*

---

[66] www.agingcare.com/discussions/thirty-percent-of-caregivers-die-before-the-people-they-care-for-do-97626.htm

When the Mount Saint Helens volcano near Olympia, Washington, began to rumble, octogenarian Harry Truman refused to leave his lodge at the foot of the volcano. Harry had led a storied life. He was a former World War I pilot and bootlegger during Prohibition.

"Damn it!" he shouted to reporters. "I'm eighty-three years old and I have the right to make up my mind and do what I want to do."

Indeed he perished when the eruption came at 8:40 a.m. on May 18, 1980, overcoming Harry, his sixteen cats, his home, his fifty-four-acre property, and all of Spirit Lake. The townspeople of Castlerock erected a memorial for their stubborn and self-determined native son.[67]

Our Story: Hits Close to Home

My dad is eighty, restores old John Deere tractors, drinks bourbon, and has two cats: a home cat and a farm cat. He does not live near a volcano, but a few years ago he did survive the *derecho* that wiped out most of his barn and part of the house. He refuses to write his will. At one point I gave up trying to reason with him. He has the right to do what he wants, but I know that someday I will be tasked with sorting out tractors, gazillions of tools, the camper, the old cars, the motorboat, the house, and more. He enjoys tinkering and can fix or repair absolutely anything, a skill I wish I had acquired but never had the interest or patience to learn. I am thrilled he fills his days with projects and socializing, a retirement routine I hope to emulate.

My mom's situation put us in a straight-up crisis mode that lasted more than a year. During the dips and downtimes of that situation, I began to bug my dad again about getting his affairs in

---

67 atulgawande.com/book/being-mortal/

order. I had learned a lot while managing my mom's situation, but my dad's was an entirely different animal.

My parents divorced when I was seven. A couple of years later, both remarried. Shortly after my mom was officially diagnosed with Alzheimer's, my stepmother was diagnosed with primary progressive aphasia, a nervous system syndrome that affects the patient's ability to speak or write or understand the spoken or written word. My stepmom, who was semiretired, had just turned seventy. I was devastated for her. She was open to exploring any therapies and suggestions to manage her new health challenge—a welcome contrast to my mom's defiant denial.

For better or worse, my stepmom had my dad to help her navigate the hard left turn leading to her future. I quickly nicknamed them "The Bickersons" because the stress of dealing with the uncertainty and behavioral changes was not easy for either of them. I phoned often to check in and began gently pushing them to get their legal and financial issues in order. When I cleaned out my mom's house, I came across books, DVDs, legal document software kits, and aging anecdotes that I boxed up and mailed to my dad and stepmom. I hoped the materials would prompt them to think about their next steps.

Phone calls can only get you so far, though. I booked a flight and told my dad I was coming for a visit to discuss matters in person and meet with an attorney. I told him to pick the attorney and make an appointment. Dad admitted he "knew a guy" from way back. Occasionally, he still saw him around town. Slightly sketchy, but it was a start. To drive the conversation forward, I wanted Dad to deal with people he was comfortable with.

The attorney's office was large and dark with an immense desk piled high with stacks of papers. The surrounding shelves were stuffed with legal manuals, photos, and tchotchkes. We settled into sturdy leather chairs opposite the desk to discuss the task at hand. The meeting was surreal but productive. I had the feeling I might be in for another wild ride but in a different direction than the one I took with my mom. The attorney set his large leather chair on a slight swivel with a subtle recline. He interspersed his estate planning advice with reminiscences about his family. We learned some things about statutory law in that state; by then my personal eldercare education spanned four different states. The attorney also gave us a few action items to follow up on—all we needed to start the process rolling.

My stepmom was very thorough in completing a comprehensive contact document. She also completed her healthcare directive and will within a few weeks. My dad, however, was still a hot mess with some of his stuff though he did compile a binder of statements and added me as a co-owner on his checking account. Progress!

He still refused to do his will, though. A jokester, he'd say, "I'm not going to die" and "The home cat inherits everything." (He admitted he loves the home cat more than me, totally fine.) I read somewhere that some people hold on to the superstition that once they complete their will, they will most certainly die sooner rather than later. I indulged his reluctance but kept coaxing him into organizing and documenting statements and accounts. He wasn't happy about it, but since he had witnessed the nightmare Mom put me through, he was somewhat sympathetic.

A few months later, I booked a second visit. That time I set an appointment with an attorney I chose. I waited until I arrived to tell Dad I was meeting with a different attorney and he was welcome to accompany me. I declared I was being responsible in trying to learn more about the process in his state so I could be prepared. I cited the Mom madness as my defense. I didn't want to be blindsided with eldercare issues again. He went with me, listened, asked questions, but still wasn't quite ready to do his will. I let it go. Patience. We all need it and, in my case, it paid off. Dad signed his will on my birthday in 2023. Best. Gift. Ever.

You can choose to work on what you can control and begin building concentric circles of care around your loved one—and yourself.

CARE COUPLE

Thirty percent of caregivers pass away before the loved one they are caring for. That number jumps even higher for spousal caregivers over seventy. They are so consumed by the demands of caregiving—and sometimes so tired of going to doctor offices—that they neglect their own health. There's a strategy to avoid such burnout and tragedy: identifying a care couple to provide a solid foundation of support.[68]

It is imperative to designate one point person to communicate, coordinate, and manage all aspects of the care plan for your parent. Recruit someone who is organized and has good communication skills to keep track of all aspects of the care plan. Understand, though, that a wingman is also needed to provide support and feedback and jump in to handle issues when the point person is overwhelmed or a situation calls for "divide and conquer" simultaneous action. Plus, some care decisions are best made with a second set of eyes, ears, and hands. Perhaps you are that point person. Perhaps you are the wingman.

Also, importantly, each member of a care couple can look after the well-being of the other.

---

68 advocateformomanddad.com/what-is-a-care-couple

CARE MANAGERS

The care couple can surround themselves with expert care—an invaluable layer of help when it comes to problem-solving, starting a care plan, and evolving it as your parent's condition and needs advance. Anyone can avail themselves of two kinds of eldercare experts. Although hiring one is an added expense, ultimately, these guides can save you money by helping you avoid expensive pitfalls and efficiently negotiate bureaucracies.

The first kind of expert, known as a consultant or certified senior advisor (CSA), can help your family decide which options are best for everyone. Though their services usually are free to the family, many times their allegiance is to a particular facility that pays them for referrals. CSAs are educated professionals, however, and they have cross-disciplinary knowledge of aging issues, problems, and solutions.

A certified senior advisor can save you time and money, especially if you don't live close to your parent or don't have time to properly research care options.[69]

The second type of expert is known as a geriatric care manager (GCM)[70] or, in recent years, life care manager. Those who fill this role are usually licensed nurses or social workers who specialize in geriatrics. They work mostly for private agencies but sometimes independently. They know the territory and guide and advocate for families caring for older relatives.

---
69 go.csa.us/
70 www.nia.nih.gov/health/what-geriatric-care-manager

When searching for a GCM, find out if they're a member of the Aging Life Care Association (ALCA).[71] Membership is only open to individuals with certain degrees and experience in human services. Only ALCA members, who follow a code of ethics, can call themselves aging life care professionals.

Geriatric care managers provide a range of duties from accompanying your parent to doctors' appointments and coordinating a care team to managing benefits, mediating family conflicts, and advocating for your parent. A GCM can see you straight through a loved one's entry into hospice care if necessary. Even then they can gently make you aware of different choices and options.

---

71 www.aginglifecare.org/

SUPPORT NETWORKS

In January 2018 I joined the Hunterdon County Chamber of Commerce to host *Happy to Help*, a weekly radio show. Each week I spent an hour interviewing an executive director, fundraiser, community champion, volunteer, or author. The goal of this volunteer endeavor was to showcase the good deeds of nonprofits in a casual, conversational way. A few months later, we began recording the show on Facebook Live.[72]

I had to shift the show schedule during fall 2021 because I was flying back and forth to LA, often to work through issues with Mom. Since I booked all the guests myself, it was easy to reschedule people or skip recording some weeks.

When we finally got Mom moved, cleaned out her house, made donations, put things in storage, sold the house, sold the car, and got everything somewhat settled, I was ready to return to my volunteer work. At that point I was immersed in reading every book I could find about dementia and Alzheimer's to better understand what we were experiencing and how I could best serve Mom moving forward.

One such book, authored by a Princeton-based eldercare consultant, came with a bookmark tucked among its pages. The bookmark displayed a quote: "Boundaries are the flip side of asking for help. And if you can do both ... if you can learn to say 'no' and 'I need your help,' you might just survive this experience." —Anne Tumlinson, Founder of Daughterhood.org.[73]

---
[72] www.facebook.com/happyhunterdon/
[73] www.daughterhood.org/

I relish an opportunity to research something that piques my interest, especially when it involves a website that ends in .org. I immediately explored every section of the Daughterhood site. The mission captivated me:

> Very few people plan for the all-encompassing role of family caregiver. When it hits, the impact affects everyone. For family caregivers, each transition comes with new challenges and opportunities for support. At Daughterhood, we strive to help family caregivers feel supported and not alone.72

I felt a Thor-sized thunderbolt of excitement shoot through me. A seismic shift was imminent from a personal, professional, and cultural perspective. With ten thousand people turning sixty-five every day, the need for this type of support network is profound.

Daughterhood Circles meet online in a casual atmosphere of camaraderie. Adults discuss challenges, share information, and evaluate possible solutions to help each other in their care journeys. To my delight, the circle coordinator accepted my request to become a circle leader. I was also fortunate to partner with a local mom and friend who had worked in the senior living industry for more than a decade. She brought a wealth of experience and knowledge to the group as well as an extensive network of consultants and contacts.

We hosted our first Zoom meeting one Wednesday evening in October 2022. Eight people signed up and five showed up on the call. I thought it went well for a first go-round.

We began by introducing ourselves and sharing a few details about our caregiving situations. We kept the conversation informal and then invited anyone to present a challenge they were currently facing as a topic for discussion. These groups are good because people are at different stages and can learn from the experiences of other caregivers who have been there and can relate. Depending on how the conversation flows and unfolds, recommendations can include websites, resources, and practical products helpful for eating, bathing, and other daily activities. The main and most poignant message is: you are not alone.

Previously, I had observed a circle call run by Rosanne Corcoran, who also moderates Daughterhood The Podcast: For Caregivers.[74] I had also participated in several helpful support group calls offered through a local elder law practice.

In all these scenarios some participants wanted answers and recommendations, some wanted to know they weren't alone, some wanted to simply vent, and others wanted to learn. I found them all very helpful.

The same could be said of AlzAuthors,[75] another informative resource for webinars and books about dementia. The first call I joined featured Patti Davis, Ronald Reagan's daughter, who wrote several books about Alzheimer's, including, most recently, *Floating in the Deep End: How Caregivers Can See Beyond Alzheimer's*.[76]

As I became more fluent in all things Alzheimer's, I contacted the Alzheimer's Association of Greater New Jersey[77] and invited them to be on the *Happy to Help* radio show.[78] Cheryl Ricci-Francione, executive director of the Greater New Jersey Chapter, brought two other people—Karen Golden, the chapter's advocacy manager, and Doreen Monks, a volunteer, advocate, and Alzheimer's patient who is also active with the Overlook Medical Center Caregivers Support Group in Summit, New Jersey. Together we conducted a well-rounded conversation about dementia, which is steadily gaining more attention everywhere.

Our talk drove home the realities of Alzheimer's and caregiving nationwide and in New Jersey. In the US six million people have Alzheimer's and someone is diagnosed every sixty-five seconds. My guests also said 190,000 New Jerseyans have Alzheimer's and 340,000 people are providing unpaid care. What an extraordinary amount of time and care and what an extraordinary number of people and medical resources. And how very much it takes for everyone, patients and caregivers, to

---

74 pod.co/daughterhood-the-podcast-for-caregivers
75 alzauthors.com/
76 www.amazon.com/Floating-Deep-End-Caregivers-Alzheimers-ebook/dp/B08X9334B2
77 www.alz.org/nj
78 www.facebook.com/happyhunterdon/videos/460273685482393

live empowered lives in their new reality.

The Alzheimer's Association itself is a lifeline for the public. Anyone who needs help can call its free helpline—800-272-3900, any day of the year.

"It's open 24-7," Golden said, "and it can be translated into two-hundred-plus languages."

Dementia patients, caregivers, family members, and the general public can speak confidentially to specialists and top clinicians, who offer support and information about symptoms, programs and services, treatment options, and legal, financial, and care decisions.

"The Alzheimer's Association is a phenomenal help," Monks said, speaking as a patient, "but there are lots of people out there who want to help you. You can have a good life. It's a different life but you can have a good life, so don't be afraid."

Also helpful are governmental units of aging services, which are called different things in different states from divisions and bureaus to commissions and departments. All are discoverable online through the Eldercare Locator.[79] These state and county resources can help caregivers navigate the system, too, and connect them with any available support services, including respite care.

---

79 eldercare.acl.gov/Public/About/Aging_Network/SUA.aspx

RESOURCES FOR FAMILIES

Advocate for Mom and Dad[80]
www.advocateformomanddad.com:

> Online community run by consultant Deb Hallisey where caregivers learn from the experiences of others.

AgingParents
www.agingparents.com:

> A consulting and conflict resolution service for families and professionals that specializes in eldercare issues. Run by a husband/wife team, one a nurse-attorney, the other a mental health professional.

Alzheimer's Prevention Registry
www.endalznow.org:

> Registry led by Banner Alzheimer's Institute that matches volunteers with opportunities to participate in their research studies.

Alzheimer Prevention Trials (APT) Webstudy
www.aptwebstudy.org:

> Study that monitors volunteers ages fifty and older for memory changes using free twenty-minute online quarterly tests.

Brain Health Registry
www.brainhealthregistry.org:

> A web-based, observational research study that captures data which helps identify and monitor cognitive changes associated with neurodegenerative diseases and brain aging.

CaringKind
www.caringkindnyc.org:

> New York City provider of programs and services for individuals with dementia, their families, and professional caregivers.

---
[80] www.facebook.com/happyhunterdon/videos/792423475347547

Community Resource Finder
www.communityresourcefinder.org:

> A database of dementia- and aging-related resources funded by the Alzheimer's Association and AARP, though the providers are not endorsed by either organization.

Conversation of Your Life (COYL)
www.njhcqi.org/coyl:

> New Jersey program that provides education and resources on how to pick a health care proxy and share your wishes for end-of-life care.

Healthy Brains
www.healthybrains.org:

> A Cleveland Clinic interactive platform that provides individualized brain health assessment tools, lifestyle tips, and medical news.

Nightingale NJ[81]
www.nightingalenj.com:

> Eldercare consulting firm that offers families eldercare navigators who help seniors and their adult children make sound choices in a confusing field of aging-related medical, financial, legal, and emotional issues.

---

81 www.facebook.com/happyhunterdon/videos/928154761436844

LIVING OPTIONS

Choosing where to live is among the biggest decisions seniors and caregivers make. In 2022 *U.S. News & World Report* looked at the most common living arrangements for American retirees: aging in place, moving in with family, house sharing, independent living, assisted living, life plan communities/continuing care retirement communities, and subsidized housing.[82] Let's explore some of these options.

AGING IN PLACE

A 2021 AARP survey shows 77 percent of adults fifty and older want to remain in their homes as they grow older—a percentage that hasn't changed for more than a decade.[83] The appeal is understandable: One doesn't lose local social networks—friends, neighbors, doctors or banks or accountants, for instance—or the comfort of a familiar environment. But the calculus of staying at home changes when the older person is cognitively impaired. Outside helpers must check in regularly. Over time other services probably will be needed, including grocery delivery, meal delivery, housekeeping, and case managers who can help with finding companions and trained caregivers.

A host of healthcare personnel can come into play and it's good to know each one's specialty and limitations:

---

[82] money.usnews.com/money/retirement/articles/housing-options-for-seniors
[83] www.aarp.org/home-family/your-home/info-2021/home-and-community-preferences-survey.html

- **Companions** do chores, prepare meals, run errands, cook, do handyman jobs, pick up (but do not administer) medications, and more. Companions are not certified.
- **Certified Nursing Aides**/Assistants (CNAs) provide hands-on care for Activities of Daily Living (ADLs) or Instrumental Activities of Daily Living (IADLs), plus companion care. CNAs are certified through a six-week course where they learn some basic medical skills, including how to check vital signs and care for wounds. ADLs include eating, bathing/showering, grooming, walking, dressing and undressing, transferring and toileting. IADLs include using the phone, shopping for groceries, making or serving meals, managing medications, cleaning, navigating transportation, and managing money. CNAs can also be called Personal Care Attendants (PCAs) or Home Health Aides (HHAs).
- **Licensed Practical Nurses** (LPNs) are licensed professionals who have completed an accredited practical nursing certificate program, usually at a community college.
- **Registered Nurses** (RNs) have a four-year bachelor's degree in nursing and have passed a state certification exam to become licensed.
- **Nurse Practitioners** (NPs) complete a graduate master's or doctoral nursing program and take a board certification exam. They can provide some of the services offered by Medical Doctors (MDs) or Physician Assistants (PAs).

All that help can be costly—concerning, too, with so many people you don't know well in the house. Of course a family member could move in with your loved one or vice versa.

Every option has pros and cons and should be carefully considered. Medicare, legal and financial issues all matter, too, and are regulated by different guidelines in different states.

If you decide to keep your parent at home as long as possible, invite a consultant to evaluate their home space for modifications that can mitigate falls and mishaps and make life more comfortable for everyone involved.

HOME SHARING

If solo aging is not an option for you or appealing to your loved one, home sharing might be a preferred alternative. Many families work out a home sharing scenario among immediate or extended family. There are also services that provide matching arrangements between older adults. Twelve million baby boomers over age sixty-five live alone, according to *Forbes*.[84]

Some areas allow adding an accessory dwelling unit (ADU) to a lot with an existing home. ADUs can be rented out to another solo ager, a college student, or a caregiver, perhaps at a reduced cost in exchange for running errands or caregiving help.[85]

NEXT GEN HOUSING

Next Gen is a home within a home that offers a separate entrance, kitchenette, living area, bedroom or multiuse room, and a bathroom.

LIFE PLAN COMMUNITIES

A Life Plan Community, or Continuing Care Retirement Community (CCRC), offers continuum-of-care options for people who want to move into a community where they can transition to more comprehensive care if their health conditions change. A resident may initially move into the Independent Living section, Assisted Living, or Memory Care, and transfer if there is space. Some newer facilities enable a loved one to move into and remain in the same room and adjust the level of care to meet their needs where they are.

A far cry from the traditional nursing home model, some modern senior living facilities resemble resorts. Their price tag resembles resort fees as well. Rates are set based on the level of care needed. Some require people to buy their unit and pay an additional monthly service or maintenance fee. Others charge a hefty monthly fee that includes most services. For even more personalized care, there are additional charges.

---

[84] www.forbes.com/sites/sarazeffgeber/2021/05/20/solo-agers-plan-now-if-you-want-to-thrive-in-later-life

[85] www.forbes.com/sites/sarazeffgeber/2021/05/20/solo-agers-plan-now-if-you-want-to-thrive-in-later-life/?sh=40c3698f7fa1

Some facilities raise rates without much notice. Read the contract carefully and ask questions.

REHAB/NURSING HOMES

Some traditional nursing homes have been rebranded as "rehabs." People who have fallen, broken a bone, or require surgery end up in rehab. These medical facilities, with skilled nurses and occupational and physical therapists on staff, are designed to be a short-term stop. Some rehab facilities offer the option of transitioning to long-term care on-site if the patient does not improve.

VILLAGE NETWORK

The village concept of living is emerging in major cities. In the context of aging, a village is a grassroots group of neighbors helping neighbors, according to Iona Senior Services, a premier aging organization in the Washington, DC, area. Paid staff run the group and often recruit volunteers to help with tasks. Each village holds its own social programs and classes. Sometimes it partners with local businesses that offer residents discounts.[86]

Starting with Beacon Hill Village[87] in the Boston area, the village concept has caught on. There are now some 350 villages in the US and worldwide. The Village to Village Network connects the Massachusetts village to all the others.[88]

Innovation in the international space offers hope for a positive evolution in dementia care that allows people to live with dignity. Examples include The Hogeweyk in the Netherlands[89] and The Village Langley[90] in Canada.

---

[86] www.iona.org/wp-content/uploads/2019/04/DC-Villages-UPDATED-2-2020.pdf
[87] www.beaconhillvillage.org
[88] vtvnetwork.org
[89] hogeweyk.dementiavillage.com/
[90] verveseniorliving.com/the-village/

WHERE TO LIVE: AN EXERCISE

How do you know which living arrangement is right for your loved one?

It's time to break out an index card and write your loved one's definition of "quality of life" in one sentence. For example, what is their joy?

On the other side of the card, write what your loved one doesn't want or is afraid of. For example, they may not want to put themselves in certain circumstances.

Conversations about where to live can be awkward. Remember, though, that choosing where to live is not about helping people die. It's about helping people live the way they want to live, with a mature life plan. Most are afraid of being in physical pain or emotional distress, being a burden on their loved ones, or not being able to leave a nugget for their loved ones. There is no universal path. We are each on our own paths. Making informed decisions while limiting risks is a win.

RESOURCES FOR HOUSING

Beacon Village
beaconhillvillage.org:

> A member-led community of independent adults age fifty and older who care for one another through an array of support services and programs.

Check for Safety
www.cdc.gov/steadi/pdf/check_for_safety_brochure-a.pdf:

> A home fall prevention checklist for older adults created by the Centers for Disease Control and Prevention and the MetLife Foundation.

The Green House Project
thegreenhouseproject.org/our-story/history:

> One hundred eldercare communities committed to providing non-institutional environments for those who live and work in them.

LeadingAge
leadingage.org/thought-leadership:

> A band of thought leaders advancing the aging process in the US.

National Family Caregiver Support Program
acl.gov/programs/support-caregivers/national-family-caregiver-support-program:

> Government programs, which vary by state, that pay family members to be a caregiver, or personal care assistant (PCA), to an elderly person to help with Activities of Daily Living (ADLs) and other tasks, such as light housekeeping and meal preparation.

Senior Advisor
www.senioradvisor.com:

> A free-to-family search and rating service that helps people find the best senior living facility for them.

Seniors Helping Seniors
seniorshelpingseniors.com:

> A franchise business that matches seniors who need help and companionship in their homes with seniors who can give help.

Silvernest
www.silvernest.com:

> A home sharing matching service for older adults.

Tracy Cram Perkins
tracycramperkins.com:

> A dementia home care specialist.

USAging
www.usaging.org:

> A vaccination coordination service across aging and disability networks.

Village to Village Network
vtvnetwork.org:

> A membership-based organization that advocates for the Village model and provides expert guidance, resources, and support to help establish and maintain thriving Villages for seniors.

THINGS TO CONSIDER: DECISION METRICS

When evaluating the best option for your loved one and your family, there are many factors to consider. To make the best decision, evaluate the following items literally and emotionally, knowing that circumstances could change and require further consideration or a different level of care as the disease progresses. Aim for peace of mind for the time being.

1. **Price:** Money is always a primary consideration, but other factors are equally important.

2. **Proximity** to family members: Having family members close by and visiting frequently can make a difference in the quality of care your loved one receives.

3. **Facility cleanliness and amenities:** Does the atmosphere appeal to you? Does it feel like a cold clinical setting or warmer like a plush hotel?

4. **Staff ratio and attentiveness:** Notice if staff is attentive to the residents or seems more focused on their phones or congregating together. Is the activities coordinator enthusiastic and engaging?

5. **Cohorts:** Are the residents cordial or contentious toward one another? Get a feel for the culture among the residents in independent living or the memory care unit. Do visitors come and go frequently or does the place feel lonely and empty?

6. **Spiritual/cultural backdrop:** Is it important to you and your family to have access to clergy or a rabbi to practice your faith? Are there other residents on-site who share your faith and level of participation and commitment? Are there other residents who speak the same native language? Many older adults revert to speaking their first language as dementia progresses.

MANAGING A MOVE

Sorting through, donating, and disposing of the contents of an entire house is unbelievably overwhelming. If you are tasked with packing up the house that you grew up in, the job can be even more challenging. In some sense most of us are hoarders. I know I am.

Where to start? You guessed it! Have the conversation. Your parent will want to feel as comfortable as possible with the move. Selecting familiar, favorite furniture and belongings will help ease the transition. They may also want to share stories about when or where they acquired certain things and who in the family they want to leave them to. A trip down memory lane may help them renew a sense of pride in what they have accomplished and make way for new experiences. Change is hard for everyone. Proceed with compassion, caution, and multiple conversations.

If you have come to the conclusion that the best step forward is to move your loved one out of their home for whatever reason, it is helpful to know there are services that can help. I found it easier to break things down and delegate where possible.

My monthly cross-country trips to LA were helpful. I could take a mental inventory of Mom's belongings by simply being in the house and opening closets and cupboards. These peeks enabled me to see what was worth keeping and research places where I could donate certain items. I tried sorting through a couple of closets with Mom, but she would insist that I was overwhelming her. She promised that she would sort on her own time and in her own way so she could be "responsible" about it all. She never acted, just talked about acting, and wouldn't allow me to touch her stuff.

Except for a few secret trunkloads, I was not able to remove and donate items while Mom was around. I contacted neighbors for recommendations on local resources, researched options, and made a list of what to tackle when Mom was napping or distracted.

The key factor to consider is time. Establish a schedule and a timeline. If you have the time and want to travel down memory lane with your loved one as you sort through family heirlooms and excavate closets, enjoy the trip! If you are under pressure to get the house cleaned out and listed in time for the spring seller's market, designate someone to do the packing and someone to take Mom away for the day while it gets done.

Estate services can assist with every aspect of this process. Decide what you prefer to hire out and what you can handle yourself. If you decide to parcel out parts of the move, make sure you understand how the fees are structured and what the company provides.

Here are some tips for dealing with just about every item in a house:

- **Shredding:** A plethora of options exist for shredding papers, so why not? Even today paper accounts for 25 percent of landfill waste and 33 percent of municipal waste.[91] Many towns host "shred days" at which you can shred for free or at minimal cost. They are very sporadic and spread out over a calendar year, so plan ahead if you can. Staples, UPS, and major chain stores typically charge one dollar per pound. It doesn't seem like much, but after we cleared out nine Bankers Boxes, it all got pretty heavy and expensive. Coupons helped reduce the cost quite a bit. I simply asked the clerk if they had any discount barcodes near the register.

- **Furniture:** Many Habitat for Humanity locations manage a ReStore where they accept and resell furniture. Sometimes they will pick up pieces at no charge, but scheduling is

---

91 legalshred.com/paper-recycling-stats-u-s/

very sporadic so, once again, planning ahead helps. I didn't have the luxury of time with the furniture, so I paid a fee to have Habitat come on a specific day and move out the large items.

- **Garage Items:** Cleaning products, paint cans, varnish, and the like are considered household hazardous waste and must be disposed of properly at a household hazardous waste facility. Some municipalities offer designated days each month or quarter to accept these items. Ask your neighbors or check Earth911 online.

- **Moving services:** If you don't have the time, energy, or patience to go through everything, hire a company that specializes in moving seniors. Some firms focus on estate sales, others on managing the move. Each one has a different level of service and fee structure. Ask friends and neighbors who they recommend. Some, such as Caring Transitions, have many locations across the United States.

- **Donations:** The Salvation Army, Goodwill, churches, and community thrift stores accept a wide range of items. They may have designated days for dropping off certain items. Some are more selective than others. Check hours of operation and confirm which categories of items are accepted or excluded before loading up the car.

RESOURCES FOR MOVING

Artifcts
artifcts.com:
> A service that offers a way to store and archive the images of, and stories behind, objects in our lives without actually saving the objects. The goal is helping people declutter without guilt.

Better World Books
www.betterworldbooks.com:
> A for-profit social enterprise and global e-retailer that diverts books from landfills by collecting them from libraries, bookstores, college campuses, and other sources with surplus materials. In so doing, it raises money for literacy. The large green donation bins of Better World Books are located primarily in the Northeast. Find the donation site nearest you at www.betterworldbooks.com/go/donate. (There are usually other local charities that collect books, too. Even your local library may take used books.)

Caring Transitions
www.caringtransitions.com:
> A franchise that provides packing, moving, and relocation services for seniors. Its locations are all across the US.

Earth911
earth911.com/inspire/safely-dispose-cleaning-products:
> A website with a database that shows how and where to dispose of household hazardous materials.

Goodwill Industries International
www.goodwillfinds.com/stores:
> A national organization whose donation drop boxes and staffed sites are ubiquitous. Goodwill accepts most gently used items.

Habitat for Humanity ReStores
www.habitat.org/restores:

Locations that accept donations and are independently owned and operated by local Habitat organizations.

National Association of Senior & Specialty Move Managers (NASMM)
www.nasmm.org:
A membership organization for move managers that has a searchable database.

Salvation Army
satruck.org:
An international charitable organization that sells donated items at their thrift stores. Proceeds fund various community programs. You can find a Salvation Army drop-off location or schedule a pickup through its website.

Smooth Transitions
www.smoothtransitions.com:
A franchise company that manages moves and estate sales nationwide.

StoryPoint Senior Living
www.storypoint.com/moving-elderly-parents-to-another-state:
A collection of senior housing communities in nine states across the US. Its website offers a plethora of advice, including creating a plan to move your parent from one state to another.

UPS Store
www.theupsstore.com/store-services/shredding:
A leading package delivery company that provides a large locked portable trash bin for shredding at its store sites. You can stuff sensitive financial documents through a slot into the bin. Shredding can be expensive, so find a coupon or ask for a discount at the register. Office supply store chains also offer such services. Additionally, many local communities schedule Senior Shred Days that provide the service free of charge.

Our Story: Living in Limbo

Nancy and Mom toured several senior facilities in the LA area multiple times. Many years earlier they had moved their mother from Iowa to LA to more closely manage her care and have her near family. Their mother did well until she fell and sustained a traumatic brain injury. She was bedridden for eighteen months until her passing. One of the residences Mom and Nancy toured was the same one their mother had lived in.

Mom went along with the idea, mostly to appease everyone else. She finally agreed on a high-end gorgeous new residence not far from where her grandsons lived. We later discovered that she had lied about putting down the deposit. We tried to work with her and allow her to call the shots because it was her life, but when we realized she was playing us, we got more aggressive with our plans and began excluding her from the conversation.

We believe Mom agreed to fly to the East Coast in January 2022 to tour senior facilities with Nancy because she felt the frustration within the family and thought that by agreeing to more tours, she could prolong the process and buy herself more time. Her trip to Maryland did not work out well.

Mom flew to Maryland with my sister to tour senior living facilities near Nancy's house. We wanted her to explore the idea of living near Nancy as we slowly coaxed her into selling her house. The financial burden and her Alzheimer's diagnosis dictated we do something soon. My sister escorted Mom to Baltimore/Washington International Airport (BWI), spent the night at Nancy's, and flew back solo to LA the next day. Nancy had set up several tour appointments at senior living centers.

The following morning my sister woke up to a text sent from Mom at 3:43 a.m. EST: "I understand that you and others have taken away my rights to my house and are cleaning it out … and it is then being sold?? And where am I to go?? Does my 'family' think that I have NO rights or that I am demented? Am I to have no say in anything? And Nancy was duplicitous in this … how cruel of everyone! I am gone!" And she was.

Nancy woke up and was trying to be quiet because she thought Mom was sleeping. She soon discovered, however, that the guest room was empty. Nancy realized Mom was missing around 8 a.m., about the same time my sister read the text. Nancy called the police, who came and filed a missing person report.

As I was waking up in New Jersey, I got texts and voicemails from Nancy and my sister. Here's the one from Nancy:

> Hello Nicole, this is your Aunt Nancy. Mom left. She packed her bags. I just came out of the room a short while ago because I got up, I got dressed, I made my bed, I thought I would not disturb her. And then I came out and realized that she was gone. Her packed bags are gone. She's gone. I just found her glasses so she obviously dropped them here. I'm guessing she went to the airport. I'm gonna go over there and see if I can find out anything to help find her. Still looking to see if she booked a flight. She said she was flying back to California so I expect that's the effort she's making and she's pretty tenacious. I thought you should know and I'll be in touch. Love you. Bye.

We checked the locator app often but Mom's phone remained dormant. I called the credit card bank and was able to access pending charges through the touchtone customer service system. I discovered she had charged a room at a national hotel chain but could not determine which location. We started calling all the properties in the Baltimore area: Baltimore/Washington International Thurgood Marshall Airport (BWI), two in Annapolis, one in Columbia, etc. There was no record of her staying at any of them.

Suddenly my sister saw Mom pop up on tracking, revealing her location at BWI. Nancy started checking airlines and flight times to Los Angeles International Airport (LAX). I called the credit card system again and discovered Mom had purchased a ticket on Southwest. Nancy alerted BWI security. They said they could monitor Mom but did not have the authority to detain her unless Nancy showed up with a durable power of attorney document, which, thankfully, she had. Nancy and her neighbor arrived at the airport, met up with security, and headed for the gate.

When Nancy approached Mom at the airport, Mom was surprised and flustered but agreed to go with them. Then she diverted and ducked into the restroom. Nancy, her neighbor, and security officers waited outside the restroom. Nancy called me quickly to let me know they were with her. Relief. Mom came out of the restroom, then went back in again. The security captain followed her into the women's restroom to retrieve her. Mom spat venomous words, grabbed Nancy's arm, and whacked her a couple of times as they were escorted back to the car. The officers closed in to protect Nancy while her neighbor tried providing moral support.

The officers stayed with them until all three were inside the car, backing out of their space, and driving away. Mom had met Nancy's neighbor before, but once they were in the car, Mom demanded to know who she was, if she was hired as a spy, and what her intentions were. This tirade continued for the duration of the ride back to Nancy's. After they arrived, Mom's demeanor suddenly shifted to one of subdued acceptance and apology. They ordered pizza and Mom recounted what she could remember of her recent escapade.

Meanwhile, I took a train from New Jersey to BWI that evening to assist Nancy in whatever would come next. When I arrived at Nancy's around 10 p.m., Mom had gone to bed for the night. Nancy filled me in on the wild adventure of the previous night. Though Mom was in the beginning stages of Alzheimer's, she was highly functional and cognizant at times. She was able to recount her recent activity, but how reliably? We will never know.

Mom explained that she knew she had to be really quiet getting out of the condo so as not to wake Nancy. She walked with her roller bag down the street at 1 a.m., wearing only a simple overcoat in thirty-degree weather. She walked and wandered around until she ran into three random guys coming out of a bar and asked them for help in giving her a ride to the airport. They obliged and dropped her at a hotel. She checked in for two nights and slept a bit, then got up the next morning and headed to BWI to book a flight. We shuddered at the notion of all that could have gone horribly wrong with her nocturnal escape.

As Nancy and I talked, Mom emerged from the bedroom asking for a washcloth or wrap because her left arm ached. Nurse Nancy examined her swollen arm and quickly determined it was a bad sprain or break. Mom did not remember injuring it. We figured she had slipped earlier when she was outside smoking. Nancy wrapped her arm and made her comfortable. Mom went back to bed. Our first stop the next day would be to urgent care for an X-ray. It was indeed broken, and casted.

Mom had had several years of gradual memory loss that went largely undetected, followed by an Alzheimer's diagnosis in July 2021, followed by six months of cross-country flights, fights, and panic attack calls. We were all exhausted and needed a plan.

We doubled down on our efforts to somehow find a permanent solution. The next step was to schedule interviews and evaluations with a couple of senior communities.

I knew the sales manager at a lovely new senior living residence less than fifteen minutes from my house in New Jersey. Several of my friends' mothers lived there. We were able to arrange two intake/assessment calls with the New Jersey residence for that very afternoon. The first Facetime with the doctor went okay despite her managing her toddler during the call—a typical scenario during COVID times. I felt like managing my own mother was like managing that toddler. We stressed over making sure she had eaten and napped before the intake interviews so she would be alert. Maybe that tactic backfired. During the doctor interview, Mom kept reiterating that she wanted to live in California and invited the doctor to visit her home and audit her bills to prove she was perfectly capable of managing her own life.

Mom did a second intake interview with a nurse and again talked constantly about her desire to continue living in sunny California and how much she loved working in the yard of her home. Mom was able to name the US president and the current month, so the nurse rejected her for consideration for the memory care unit at their facility. We were back to square one.

Nancy and I stopped caring if Mom overheard us openly discussing "where we are going to put her." We were exhausted, annoyed, and at our wits' end. We discussed our legal and psychiatric options for moving forward.

Frustration levels were flying high again as we grew tired of the flux in plans and her mood swings, demands, and defiance. Mom outlined how she would take control: if she was doomed to live in a facility, she would refuse to eat until she wasted away to nothing. She was terrified of becoming lost and withdrawn. She and Nancy had witnessed the recent gradual deterioration of their oldest sister, who was suffering from vascular dementia and lived with her daughter in the Midwest.

I call Mom "the chameleon." She can be a maniacal lunatic, mean and vicious, and then completely calm and rational to anyone she perceives is evaluating her. I learned later that paranoia and personality shifts can be symptoms of the disease.

Mom's "right to die" mantra was a frequent one. She complained it would be much easier to have cancer. She never anticipated getting Alzheimer's disease. She said her life had been good and she was more than ready to die and be with Bert, my stepfather. She said she "was somebody" once and she didn't have anything left to do.

My friend sent information about a psychiatric hospital in New Jersey. Nancy spoke with their director of mental health, who listened to our predicament and concern. She advised on how a direct admission could come from a hospital emergency department. They could then admit Mom to the psych facility and keep her a couple of weeks to evaluate her, issue meds, if necessary, and get her stabilized.

Before we resorted to that option, Nancy wanted to visit one more place the following day.

The next morning, we drove to an established, well-respected mental health, special education, developmental disability, and social services hospital in the Baltimore area. Nancy was hoping Mom would voluntarily admit herself.

Mom had always dealt with depression and took medication for it, so we worried that her condition might be exacerbating her behavior. We still weren't sure how much of her erratic behavior could be attributed to Alzheimer's or whether additional anxiety and psychosis factors were at play. Nancy attempted to fill out the paperwork but Mom hastily snatched it away and made a commotion in the waiting room. She wanted to take control of the situation and clearly communicated her disapproval to everyone. The receptionist was adept in handling her complaints and outbursts of indignation at being there.

They took Mom and Nancy back to the nurse practitioner to speak about Mom's current state of mental health. They invited her to agree to a voluntary hospital admission. She refused.

I did not look forward to the drive home that evening. I'm not sure I even realized what we would do next, but Nancy advised me to drive back to New Jersey with Mom and go directly to the emergency room at the hospital near my house. My daughter, who was visiting friends in Maryland, would accompany us back to New Jersey. Her presence was a huge comfort to me. Otherwise, I might have gone mad.

Mom stayed mostly quiet and brooded in the back seat as we made our way from Maryland to New Jersey on that gloomy gray day. My daughter quietly played her music. I tried to remain calm but the closer we came to the hospital, the more my anxiety mounted. I knew that when Mom realized what we were up to, a confrontation would erupt. I briefly considered stopping by the house for a night or two and letting her settle and rest after a weary week, but I knew it was now or never. We had to figure out what was driving her behavior, even if it all seemed a bit dramatic. I trusted Nancy completely in her medical knowledge and navigation of the system and I knew she would only do what was best for her sister. We had exhausted all other avenues.

Conservatorship was front and center in the national news in 2021, the same time we were dealing with our dementia dilemma with Mom. The #FreeBritney campaign was in full swing to allow pop star Britney Spears to end the conservatorship under which her father controlled her personal life, finances, and medical decisions. Ultimately, Britney prevailed. Her conservatorship had two parts: one for her estate, one for her person. Mom had all her legal documents in place, but our efforts to convince her to move were going nowhere. We discussed the option of conservatorship at length with the elder law attorney. He advised that this route might be the only way to remove Mom from her house. We were simultaneously pursuing several plans, both in California and New Jersey, conservatorship being the last resort. We'd been hoping to put Mom's house on the market after the first of the year, and she was nowhere closer to making a plan to live elsewhere.

Several months prior, as the holiday season got underway, Nancy and I had discussed all options in detail. I failed to understand one critical fact: once we agreed to go the conservatorship route and get the initial court date, it could be another five months before we could legally and forcibly remove Mom from the house. *Five months?!* Here we were in January in crisis mode. We could not endure another five months of insanity and uncertainty.

ACUTE INCIDENT

Many elders end up in the emergency room (ER) due to a fall or because their vitals are not where they should be or a concerned family member or caregiver notices something is off. If a person is admitted to the hospital for care, the primary goal is treatment, followed by a quick discharge. Hospitals are incentivized to discharge patients. They are also penalized for too many readmissions. Various staff specialists coordinate the care and plan for the patient. It's good to know how to navigate the emergency room.

Whether arriving via ambulance or as a voluntary "walk-in," patients wait in the designated ER admission area until they are evaluated and then, depending on the nature and severity of their medical issue, possibly admitted to the hospital.

Clerical and technical personnel gather personal information and take vitals to create a record in the system. Eventually a nurse will conduct an evaluation, followed by a physician. A specialty physician may be summoned to see the patient in the ER, or the patient could be admitted to the hospital to whatever unit is required for adequate care—orthopedics, surgery, cardiology, psychiatry, intensive care, etc.

MEDICAL PROFESSIONAL STAFF DIRECTORY

It's helpful to know the roles and responsibilities of those who work in an ER:

- A **hospitalist** is a medical doctor with the same education and training as your primary care physician but with a specialty in providing care for patients in a hospital setting.[92]

- A **physician advisor** coordinates among different departments, teams, and staff involved with patient care. They are liaisons whose job is to ensure compliance with all hospital regulations.

- A **geriatrician** is a primary care doctor with additional training in treating older adults, especially those sixty-five and up.

- A **gerontologist** has patients but is not a medical doctor. The title applies to all experts in the field of gerontology, which is the study of aging and its effects on medical treatment and well-being.

- A **physician assistant** (PA) holds a graduate degree and requires a state exam for registration. They can provide roughly 80 percent of the duties an MD can perform, which can include diagnosing, ordering and evaluating tests, treating, and writing prescriptions. However, a PA can only deliver services under the license of a specific doctor.

- A **doctor of osteopathic medicine** (DO) is a fully trained and licensed doctor who has attended and graduated from a US osteopathic medical school. Traditional doctors of medicine (MDs) graduate from a conventional medical school.

- A **discharge planner** is usually a nurse who facilitates the process after the physician signs off. Nurses are your friends, right through the end of your hospital stay. In any institutional situation, find out who the primary nurse

---

92 www.webmd.com/a-to-z-guides/what-is-a-hospitalist-doctor

is. Who else is in charge? How do rounds work? Express genuine gratitude for care and ask questions. It's easier to escalate an issue when there is a perceived problem if you are polite and know something about the process. People want to do their jobs well, but nobody likes a nag.

DISCHARGE ORDERS

Congratulations, your loved one has been discharged. What's next?! Where do you go? There are many options:

- **Home:** Most patients go home.

- **Acute Rehab:** An inpatient rehab facility where an MD visits daily and a team of professionals align and integrate for a patient's treatment goals. These specialists can include physical therapists, occupational therapists, and speech therapists.

- **Skilled Nursing Facility (SNIF):** A facility whose staff includes medical doctors (MDs) and nurse practitioners (NPs). When they work in a SNIF, these two medical professionals are sometimes called "SNIFists."

- **Subacute Rehab:** A rehab facility a level lower than acute rehab in terms of intensity, the patient's condition, and rehab efforts.

- **Long-term acute care hospital** (LTACH): Essentially a hospital within a hospital where an MD visits daily. A LTACH is similar to a subacute facility but affords easier access to specialists, such as internists, pulmonologists, and respiratory therapists.

TAMING THE BULL

Defending their independence, your parent may become difficult to help and resistant to change. They might casually discourage you from dropping by because they don't want you seeing the layers of dust on the furniture and lack of food in the icebox. They may have forgotten to take their meds or skipped picking up refills. But even if their situation hasn't reached such extremes, your parent may need assistance and yet fiercely refuse any.

At these times remember their overall situation and the life adjustments they're being forced to make. They don't like them any more than you do. As we age, we are forced to relinquish certain things we take for granted, including driving. That's a difficult pill to swallow, more so for some than for others. When you talk to your parent, use the word "I" versus the accusatory "you," the one exception being "I love you."

Also, dementia can come with paranoia, causing a loved one to see your interventions and attempts to help as an invasion of their privacy. Some often accuse family members of stealing things—golf clubs, money, documents, anything. Any attempt to reason with your loved one can quickly escalate into frustration.

The path of least resistance is to agree with them and meet them in their current reality. People with dementia easily lose track of time, which day of the week it is, or the current season. To communicate best with them, keep watching and waiting for the best moments.

Difficult family dynamics can compound the situation and quickly become exponentially exasperating when a health crisis occurs. Scheduled conversations and open communication are key in managing the situation. Much easier said than done.

Some family members have always been difficult to deal with and will continue that pattern. Parents may be somewhat resilient but get grouchy and combative as aches and pains and other challenging aging issues bombard them.

Our Story: Plan C

As we pulled into the lot for the hospital emergency room in New Jersey, Mom quickly realized we were not at my house and said so. She became alert and angry after the long car ride. She was also craving another cigarette. I briefly told her she was being evaluated again. After the doctor visit for the wrist debacle and the contentious interview that morning in Baltimore, she was not happy to be at yet another facility. She glared at me from the back seat.

"What are you doing to me now, bitch?!"

My eighteen-year-old daughter was stunned and embarrassed, but I told her to follow her grandmother as she went off to smoke while I waited in line for admission to the emergency room. Omicron was spiking, so the hospitals were quite busy again. My husband showed up so my daughter could go home. Mom has always been fond of my husband, but he has never liked conflict or drama, and this situation was high on both. I thanked him for coming. He shrugged and smirked to express his support and discomfort. Mom shook her cigarette at him.

"So you're in on it too, eh?" she said. "Of course you are."

I gave her intake information to the nurse/tech who motioned for Mom to come forth. Mom stopped at the security desk, just outside, and cried and complained to the guard that her family was betraying her. The admissions nurse called her over, took her vitals, and got us checked in. Due to COVID-19, multiple signs read "NO VISITORS PATIENTS ONLY," but the staff realized Mom was an exception and allowed me to stay with her. She muttered her disdain, paced around the waiting room, and headed to the bathroom while I waited outside.

The elder law attorney happened to call from California to see how things were going. When Mom came out of the bathroom, she saw me on the phone, which set her off again. She was constantly paranoid we were all talking about her (we were) and making plans for her (we were). She got in my face.

"Get away!" I yelled at her.

The staff called her name. It was her turn to be seen. Mom was still annoyed with me and strongly expressed that I not be allowed to come with her. The staff instructed me to come but asked me to keep my distance. They stuck me in an alcove around the corner while Mom waited to be evaluated. I cautiously peeked around sporadically to check on her. Sometimes she would catch me looking and return my gaze with her most venomous glare. I think she took slight comfort in knowing I was there but made it clear I would pay.

The hallway was lined with beds. A constant stream of EMTs, nurses, techs, physicians, custodians, and gurneys galore navigated the narrow hallway/highway. Phones rang. Machines beeped. Purposeful bodies in scrubs stood among patients with solemn faces enduring pain and discomfort, silently suffering, awaiting attention. I was struck by the buoyant buzz and cheerful disposition of most staffers I observed, particularly because news reports claimed COVID-19 continued to dominate and overwhelm the hospital system and staff everywhere.

One man lay comfortably on his side, snatching snoozes, looking relaxed and calm with an oxygen apparatus strapped around his head and face. He evoked an air of familiarity and seemed to be a frequent flyer in these parts. He was friendly with the staff and offered empathetic advice as he watched our dysfunctional mother/daughter dynamic unfold.

"I am a family therapist," he said. "Good luck!"

As we waited, Mom got agitated and anxious. There wasn't much room and she was clearly a wander risk, so the staff kindly asked her to stay in place. She seemed scared and seething but also somewhat aware that if she acted out, she'd risk being immediately admitted. She calmed down momentarily and focused on a random wall poster. Was that a short reprieve to process what may be happening to her? A return to reality—and anger—followed. Indignation would resurface and she would make her presence and opinion known to anyone within earshot.

I talked with the nurse, resident, and attending physician. They spoke with me separately in hushed tones around the corner from Mom. I relayed the events of the previous week that had led us to the emergency room. Mom demanded privacy when they spoke with her, so they had to set up a trifold screen around her hallway bed during discussions. Mom had run a healthcare consulting company for a decade and was well aware of, and very vocal about, rights and regulations under the Health Insurance Portability and Accountability Act of 1996 (HIPAA).

Mom wandered over to wash her hands in a random sink in the hallway, which happened to be near my corner hideout. I was talking with the attending physician at the time, who immediately cautioned Mom about getting her cast wet. When Mom realized I was there and talking about *her* to the doctor, she demanded to be part of the conversation. The attending distracted her and said she would circle back around to chat with me. The nurse was wary as to whether they would be able to get Mom into patient scrubs for eval and admit but, after much protest from Mom, they got it done. They eventually found her a room and someone to keep an eye on her. They instructed me to go home and wait.

I did not want to leave but felt my presence was inciting Mom's anger. If I stayed, I would make things more difficult for the staff, so I left. They said she would most likely be there all night and most of the next day, too. I had no idea she would be there an entire week!

The wait at home was agonizing. Every time I passed her roller bag sitting in the mudroom, a pang of guilt came over me. It felt awful and surreal to be home and know she was stuck in a sterile, windowless room alone, just fifteen minutes away. She called and said she'd lost her purse. Should I have taken it with me? I placed a frantic call to the nurses' station and they explained the purse probably was locked up per standard protocol upon admittance. I called the hospital and the mental health line every six to eight hours for updates and questions about how the process would unfold.

Mom had to be evaluated by mental health professionals, then a psych doctor, then a rep from a care facility, then psych again. All these visits would take place according to the schedules of the doctor, staff, and hospital—not Mom's—so it took time.

Our Story: Transfer to Psychiatric Hospital

The morning after Mom was admitted to the emergency department, the crisis center counselor called me. He said that Mom's initial evaluation and discussion went well and that she presented well. He didn't understand why she had been admitted.

"She seems normal," he said.

Apparently, the gerontologist also met with Mom at some point. No feedback there.

I emailed the counselor the lack of capacity letters from Mom's California doctors, the witness account from Nancy's neighbor regarding the BWI police escort incident, and a brief narrative history from our observations of Mom's behavior over the last couple of years. That seemed to change his diagnosis.

The next day the psych department saw Mom. The initial eval from psych determined that Mom presented well. They wanted to know why she was in the emergency department. Again, I relayed past events, self-harm threats, and examples of lack of clarity and ability. The tech assured me she would add my notes to the file.

Mom easily had the crisis health and psych doctor believing that she was perfectly fine and that her presence in the emergency department was preposterous. She made demands and a commotion the night she was admitted. But the attending physician, who was from Maryland, didn't take much convincing. She said she was familiar with the psych facility we had visited earlier that day in an attempt to get Mom to admit herself. The attending physician might have had more experience in dealing with dementia-related behaviors than most.

I emailed additional patient reports from Mom's California patient portal to the hospital team. Mom was eventually moved to the psych emergency department "blue zone" for further assessment and holding. There they took away her cell phone. We provided two phone numbers, mine and Nancy's, in case Mom wanted to call us. She talked to Nancy and me several times during her stay there.

Mom said she was bored, lonely, annoyed, and repeated all the familiar mantras, including "I am going back to live in my house." Her agitation probably was heightened by the fact she couldn't smoke in the hospital though she didn't specifically mention that.

She was very upset that they took her phone. It may have been a blessing, though, because she often reread old texts and emails and got worked up over things that were no longer relevant. I hated to think of her so unhappy and cooped up. She wasn't aware of time or even what day it was—a consistent lapse in her memory for months. She was in a room without windows, but she did have a TV.

Two days later the screener from a local psych hospital went to Mom's room at 2 a.m. to evaluate her but she was asleep. Go figure. Nurses had given her an Ativan injection to calm her. The screener interview finally transpired sometime early that evening. We waited on a second psych eval.

The next day the crisis center indicated they would issue a certification for involuntary admission for a psych facility transfer. But we'd have to wait on a second psych eval before they would release her.

The time between calls to the hospital for status updates was agonizing. I was calling various professionals about what our options would be and preparing for what felt like infinite "if scenarios" that could play out at the end of Mom's hospital stay.

The cast on her wrist continued to confuse her. She didn't recall injuring herself or the visits to urgent care or the orthopedist. She complained about her wrist being sore but was adamant that it was time for the cast to come off. The wrist had been casted three days earlier. Yet she insisted it had been three weeks. Mom said she had injured her wrist working in the yard. To me, the bone break and casting were a physical manifestation of the recent turn of events and her state of mind.

In addition to the dementia, we all felt there was a psychotic component to Mom's behavior that needed to be assessed and addressed. Her history of depression may have played a large role in her mental health decline in addition to the developing dementia. We were advised that the only path to an involuntary psych admission for those over age sixty-five was through a medical ER visit.

The hospital sent out referrals to psych facilities. We waited to hear back on availability. Meanwhile, Mom's will remained ironclad and her commitment to manipulation and control did not wane. She kept attempting to wield guilt and authority over those of us desperately trying to protect her assets and transition her into a safe environment with others.

Mom remained hyperfocused on her California life, her neighbors, and her friends. In reality, she had one friend she saw occasionally. Yet she had cancelled the last two outings with said friend.

Faithfully, she kept saying the same things: "I am returning to my house," "I pay all my bills," "I will go through my things and give them away," "I have an attorney and a team working with me; I am doing it," "I am sorry I vented to my family and I will not talk to you anymore," "I can drive my car, but I don't drive it much anymore anyway," "I have memories in my house and I do not need to move," "My monthly expenses are seven thousand per month and the new place is the same cost, so I will just stay where I am," "I have plenty of money to do as I choose."

At this juncture we were hoping we could drop the option of pursuing conservatorship. It would be lengthy, costly, and messy if we had to wait many months for the justice system to do its thing to allow us to forcibly remove Mom from her home. Nancy and I could not fathom six more months of Mom madness. We hoped we could go the alternate route and prayed that the referral for admission to a psych facility would come through.

Six agonizing days after arriving in the emergency room, Mom was transported by ambulance to a geriatric psychiatric program that specializes in the diagnosis and treatment of depression and Alzheimer's disease. The hospital never notified us about the transfer.

I found out when a woman from the program called me because there was a discrepancy in Mom's file, specifically the chart notes, which mentioned her fractured arm and cast. Mom showed up without a cast and nobody could explain when or how it was removed?!

Mom spent several weeks in the psych hospital with a physician who was able to evaluate her and stabilize her manic moods and depression through moderate medication. They kept us informed of her care and she was able to call us occasionally. With her safely stabilized and in a facility, we were able to focus on clearing the house for sale.

Our Story: Psych Hospital to Senior Living

Mom was being discharged from the psych hospital directly to a memory care facility. Nancy had found a brand new fabulous place just fifteen minutes from her house. The plan was for my husband and me to pick Mom up and drive her down to Maryland, but we had no idea how Mom would react.

My husband and I drove to get Mom. It was relatively warm for February. At least we had bright clear sunshine to navigate our way to Maryland that day.

After we reached the psych hospital and announced our arrival on the intercom, several staffers passed Hubby and me as we waited under the green awning for Mom to be released. One nurse commented that I looked just like my mother. I was relieved we had made it that far. After several weeks in the program, Mom would be reunited with us and securely moved into her new place. Whether she would even get out of the car once we arrived in Maryland was an unknown in the equation. Her transfer had been mandated in the release paperwork, though, and we would go with those instructions.

A nurse appeared with two brown paper bags containing Mom's belongings. I had sent the clothes, cards, and puzzles.

There were also a few sticky notes with our phone numbers and some personal hygiene items. The staff asked if her arm brace was in the bags. It wasn't. We had been told that, upon her arrival, she had been taken to the ER to get a new cast. Evidently not.

Finally, Mom appeared at the door. She walked out and right into my outstretched arms. I enveloped her as rivulets of tears streamed down her cheeks and disappeared behind her blue surgical mask. I silently sobbed with her. The nurse, dressed in blue scrubs, was there with her discharge folder. He had a muscular physique and a pleasant smile. I had spoken to him on the phone shortly after Mom arrived. He had helped find some puzzles for her to work on before our personal care packages arrived. He wasn't much taller than Mom. He wished Mom well and made sure we understood that "she really prefers to live in California" before he disappeared behind the double doors.

After all we had been through and where we were headed, I didn't appreciate being told what Mom wanted. What she wanted wasn't financially, legally, or physically feasible at that point!

Mom was in a state of slight wonder that she was finally free. She requested we head directly to a drugstore to purchase some chocolate. I already had a stash of chocolate almonds and gummy bears for her in the car. I sat in the back seat with her. She asked for tissues and cried quietly for a bit.

"Are we going to your house for just one night?" she asked. I wasn't sure if she was still capable of plotting an escape, or simply wanted to be somewhere that was somewhat familiar. I avoided the question as my husband hit the highway and headed south.

I didn't force small talk or any talk at all. No need for questions or rehashing what happened unless she wanted to discuss anything. She dove into the almonds a bit, then asked how "all of this" happened. I summarized the basic scenario of her late-night wandering and the events that followed in a few short sentences delivered in a calm, subdued tone.

Mom chose to direct her ire at Nancy. I think she knew we were headed to Maryland. She kept saying, "She did this" and "She thinks she controls my life and has all the power." I reminded her we made decisions by a group consensus with her input. I told her we were working her plan and had tried for more than a year to help her move but that she had refused over and over again.

"Your random escape in the middle of the night endangered you," I explained. "It frightened us all into action."

As we progressed down the bland, boring New Jersey Turnpike, flanked by warehouses, dead trees, and not much else, Mom commented on the dismal scenery that was so very different from the landscape she knew and loved in vibrant, verdant California. Sigh.

After a quick stop at the Joe Biden rest area in Delaware, we continued our trek southward.

As we got closer, Mom cried steadily and silently. She refused my offering of more tissues. I let her be. She had been through a lot. And, from her perspective, her lot wasn't going to get much better. We exited the highway and looped around to see the substantial senior living building come into view.

"So it's a church?!" Mom asked. The building, crowned with a cupola, was newly built and had a covered circular drive at the entrance. To me it resembled an upscale hotel, typical of the newer senior care facilities that are sometimes referred to as "cruise ship" living.

We parked and I went in to find Nancy. I had been texting her updates along the way. My husband stayed with Mom because she refused to get out of the car. Big surprise. I wasn't going to push it. I met a few staff members in the lobby and hoped they would know how to handle this scenario. They gave me a quick intro and overview and handed me a panic watch for Mom to wear.

"There's no way she'll agree to wearing that," I said. They acquiesced.

Shane, a friendly staff member, escorted me upstairs to see Mom's room. I was encouraged by the abundance of natural light, alcoves for gathering, tasteful décor, and the overall feeling of comfort, warmth, and welcome.

As Shane escorted me into the memory care unit, a slight bald man became my first random resident acquaintance. He wore tennis shoes, black track pants, and a long-sleeved forest green button-down shirt with a golf course logo. He wasn't smiling, but he wasn't scowling either. He made expectant, direct eye contact. A friend in the business had explained to me that the population in memory care units varies widely among senior residence communities. I wondered if my first acquaintance was the norm or an anomaly. I knew Nancy had vetted the place and was impressed.

Shane led me to Nancy in Mom's room. Nancy had been watching from the window, which overlooked the parking lot. I told her she was the current target of Mom's anger and blame.

Then Shane and I returned to the car where Mom was still sitting in the back seat. I introduced her to Shane whose help I had enlisted to coax her upstairs.

"I'm sure you're a nice man," she said, "but I want no part of this."

He was gracious and pleasant. Mom must have realized she was outnumbered and there was nowhere for her to go, so she eventually followed us into the building and up to her room. Nancy greeted her with a big sister hug. Mom's temporary anger melted away in the embrace.

The room was outfitted with temporary furniture until the moving company brought Mom's things. The memory care unit director was wonderful and assured us she would help Mom feel welcome. We were advised not to linger, to let Mom settle in. She immediately retreated to the corner of the bathroom and cried. I wanted to cry, too. I had suffered in uncertainty while Mom progressed through the wards in the emergency room. I picked up every time she called with her panicked pleas from the psych facility. I sorted, packed, donated and stored everything from her house in LA. It had been a hellacious four weeks. Finally, she was where she would be safe and well cared for in the best of all possible scenarios. The ordeal was very hard on all of us. I trusted the director and took her advice. We left.

Nancy and I went back to her place to decompress. We were still in shock that the entire situation was possibly settled, but far from over. A couple of hours later, Nancy's phone rang. Her cousin Brenda in California was calling. Mom had wasted no time calling people on her cell phone to relay how her sister and her daughter had unjustly shipped her to a nursing home. Brenda said Mom spent an hour on the phone, sobbing in disbelief about why and how all of this could have happened. Brenda was clearly alarmed, but Nancy explained our side of the saga. Brenda, who lived in LA, had connected with Mom and Nancy occasionally. She had visited Mom once during the pandemic when they spent a lovely day on the back patio catching up. Mom was adept at casual conversation, so it was unlikely Brenda noticed anything amiss with her memory.

Nancy and I were fine with Mom calling anyone she felt would listen to her. We also knew nobody could relate to what we had endured the past year.

While packing up the house, I had collected the holiday cards and letters Mom had received. Now that she was somewhat settled, I wrote to a few people I vaguely knew because Mom had mentioned them over the years. I shared Mom's new address and a brief summary of her diagnosis, along with my information if they wanted to know more.

In one letter we found, Mom wrote fondly of a colleague at the University of Iowa who had helped her navigate campus life and gave her the confidence to pursue every dream.

> I was twenty-nine and divorced when my life really began. I made a decision to seriously pursue a full program at the university and went about searching out just how I would do that, given the restraints of kids, money, time, etc. I met with a woman through Career Services and Planning at the University of Iowa, Tara. She was amazing and to this day must receive enormous credit for helping me learn what it truly meant to "get where I wanted to go"! Tara really listened to me and she mapped out a plan of action responsible for letting me know what I COULD DO, not what I could not do.
>
> With her knowledge and willingness to help, I moved to my college town with my three kids, got an apartment, got a full-time college schedule and a part-time work schedule that allowed me to come and go to class during the day so I could also be home with my kids most of the time.
>
> —9/97

I also discovered a wonderful framed picture of Mom and Tara. I have many childhood memories of Friday night pizza dinners with Tara and her husband at The Green Pepper in Coralville. They had always been dear friends. I mailed the picture frame to Tara with my phone number. A week later I got a concerned callback. Coincidentally, Tara lived just an hour from Mom's senior living facility and began visiting Mom weekly. A true miracle.

Mom often commented that she rarely heard from Nancy or me but always looked forward to and remembered visits from Tara. Meanwhile, Nancy visited four to five times each week and I was there every couple of weeks. Yet we were easily forgettable! Tara's father suffered from dementia, so she was intimately familiar with the disease and deeply aware of what Mom was going through. We are beyond blessed to have her friendship and frequent visits.

Mom and Tara had been part of a foursome who worked together at the University of Iowa. Even after they scattered to different parts of the country, they kept in close touch through the years. They gathered every few years for weekend getaways. Mom had her three gal pals, and her three sisters, as circles of comfort and carefree fun. She and my stepdad had had an active social life as a couple, too. They were out and about every Saturday night without fail. Though she lost her husband, confidant, and best friend when he passed away in 2002, the strong sisterhood and good friendships had remained solid and sustained her over the years. They were an anchor of stability as Mom's world changed around her.

"I WANT TO GO HOME"

Once you have evaluated all the options, made the decision, and moved your loved one into a safe space, you may hear them express the desire to "go home." Some seniors in memory care frequently and creatively pack up belongings using garbage bags or some other handy vessel to prepare to move back home. But, of course, they are packing in vain.

For a person who has dementia, the word "home" cannot necessarily be interpreted literally. If they are in an assisted living or memory care community, they may reference their old house as "home" or, as time goes on, even the address where they grew up.

Sometimes, though, "home" may be more of a feeling, or, as the Alzheimer's Society phrases it, "the sense of home rather than home itself."[93]

People with dementia can also tend to wander. Around 2009, to reduce wandering, fake bus stops were introduced in the corridors or gardens of some nursing homes in Germany. They were made to look real, featuring information boards, timetables, and even bus stop signs, all fake. A bus will never arrive. This idea proved controversial and has sparked ongoing ethical debate.[94]

The central issue, though, is a person with dementia struggling to feel a sense of belonging and familiarity while, all the time, snippets of memory come and go. The struggle is especially real if they are adjusting to a new environment—new surroundings, new people, new routines, new smells, new sensory overload. Take that unmistakable feeling of being unsettled, add a dose of suspicion, paranoia, and a sense of betrayal, and you've got a state of mind—not one we usually associate with "home." Now combine those feelings with a heightened sense of anxiety as your family members, attempting to boost your morale, paste smiles of positivity on their faces and exclaim, "Welcome to your new home!" Yikes.

Most professionals involved with eldercare and working in senior living facilities are familiar with these feelings and challenges and help make the transition easier. As mentioned, my mother initially spent many hours crying in the bathroom. We stocked a healthy supply of tissue boxes. It sounds horrible, and it is, but a tough emotional transition is inevitable. I didn't like admitting my mom was literally locked up in memory care, but knowing she was safe was better than constant worry and suicide threats from three thousand miles away.

---

[93] www.alzheimers.org.uk/blog/i-want-go-home-what-to-say-to-someone-in-dementia-care

[94] ijhpr.biomedcentral.com/articles/10.1186/s13584-019-0301-0

Moving and change is difficult for most people, at any age, even under the best of circumstances. Creating a comforting environment with favorite and familiar items, such as clothing, furniture, photos, and food, may help their transition. Take the time to listen, confirm, and validate their feelings, understanding the whole time that their desire to go "home" may be more of a pining for a sense of security and control over their life. Remember that they no longer reside in rational thinking or your reality. They live in a new, personal version of isolated reality that they don't quite understand and yet adamantly defend.

Mom moved into memory care in February 2022, shortly after her seventy-seventh birthday. The initial few weeks were difficult, followed by a flood in the facility that required another temporary move that really confused her. Months and months later, her mantra remained the same. We talked almost daily about when she'd be able to find somewhere else to move to. Here's a typical voice mail from Mom:

> Hi Nicole, it's already late today but call me tomorrow or something if you can. I'm in this place, which is nice and a facility. I'm not gonna continue to stay here and I've got to talk. ... I just want to talk it through and then I'm gonna leave.

She constantly mentioned the need to move to a place where she could be more socially active. We explained to her that she was in a place where she was surrounded by residents, staff, and family and that it was the best environment for her and her brain. Instead she envisioned herself moving to a community apartment complex where she'd return to her daily routine of going to the grocery store and conversing with neighbors on occasion. She refused to believe or admit that her memory issues prevented her from living alone.

We constantly reassured her, through reasoning, that she was where she needed to be, but we had to get better about validating and redirecting so she felt heard and comforted, not constantly corrected.

Our Story: Baby Stalking

We come from a giant Irish Catholic family full of expression, emotion, and an unbridled love of babies. My mother and her five siblings procreated and adopted to produce twenty-one first cousins.

Mom was always feisty and fostered a need to break free from the guilt-ridden confines of Irish Catholic school indoctrination. She was bent on raising hell even if it destined her to damnation. Her bravado was grounded in the secure, loving, safe, and familiar town/school/parish community where she grew up. That support and those surroundings provided her a strong foundation to launch from.

Mom embraced the women's movement even though she was saddled in suburbia with three small kids. She always wanted babies and adored them. Yet she also desperately wanted to pursue a career when she saw professional pursuits for women expand beyond the traditional roles of nurse, nun, and teacher. She found a way to do it all, as many of her peers did at that time, without agonizing over choices or feeling crippled by guilt. She had endured enough Catholic guilt to bother with the guilt that haunts so many moms today.

I love babies, too. After college graduation, I worked full-time but spent my Saturday afternoons in the labor and delivery department at a local hospital, holding babies and gossiping with the nurses. This was well before the lockdown days when, for good reason, hospital security got seriously intense. I absolutely adore babies but knew I wanted to have a career and wait for the right guy, so my volunteer endeavor appeased my baby craving without sacrificing sleep or requiring me to honor the other monumental commitments that come with raising little creatures!

It was worth the wait. I got married about a decade later and had five healthy babies and four miscarriages. I am beyond blessed.

Mom got upset when I chose to leave the workforce and stay home to raise our kids. Because she had fought hard to earn her degree while raising us, she saw me as a traitor. I reasoned that the efforts of progressive women had given me the gift of choice. I had the luxury of choice and I made mine.

We got Mom somewhat settled in the senior residence and made it a point to partake in happy hour, scheduled on-site in the "pub" at 3:30 every afternoon. Mom was never a big drinker, but Nancy and I enjoy our adult beverages immensely, so we enthusiastically attend whenever we visit. Occasionally, we get a glimpse of Maisy, the famous "baby on campus"! She is the grandbaby of a resident. Her father proudly parades her around or zips through the hallway on his mother's mobility scooter while Maisy gleefully beeps the horn. Mom lights up immediately at the sight of Maisy and follows the little one's every move.

We began our baby stalking outings almost immediately as we explored the area around Mom's new address. We walked through the nearby mall, which was full of strollers and toddlers and babies galore. The mall has a designated play space surrounded by a small wall where we can watch with delight as the kids run wild as their parents scroll their phones. We also found a nearby playground that is pretty popular and full of families. The café at the local Whole Foods has a steady stream of families coming and going, too.

On Halloween I took Mom to baby story time at the local library to see all the littles in their costumes attempting to sit still. We sat on chairs in the back with another woman. She explained she was the mother of the librarian conducting story time. It wasn't long before my mom was on the floor making faces and having fun with a tiny tot.

I often comment and explain to the wary parents that we just enjoy watching babies. Some are proud and anxious to show off their prodigy, some are wary, and others simply too exhausted to care. Some are more comfortable when I share that I have five of my own and I am biding my time until they are old enough to produce grandchildren.

Mom and I have found something fun and meaningful we can frequently do together. Mom is best when she can truly live in the moment, free of worry and searching for what she has lost and can't remember or can't find. She and the toddlers are in the same frame of mind and Mom can experience the joy of discovery they openly display on their chubby little faces.

Try to find something your loved one enjoys doing that will immerse them in the moment. Music is a good place to start. Turn on the radio, play a favorite album, or attend a local concert performed by a high school choir or professional orchestra.

Our Story: Safe but Bored

Mom is safe. Mom is bored. What do we do now? When she lived alone, she was lonely but she had previously established routines in her home that kept her settled. She played her favorite music and always had a puzzle working on the kitchen table. In hindsight I noticed she rotated three specific puzzles—a Hershey candy compilation, Ruth Bader Ginsburg, and desert cacti. The interlocking images consumed her days, which was good. Over the years she had collected about one hundred puzzles. We made sure to pack twenty or so to accompany Mom to her new home in memory care. Once she got situated, though, she stopped doing puzzles altogether. I bought her a special puzzle table that fit perfectly in her room and got one going. She never touched it. When she called to tell me she was bored, I asked her about doing the puzzle and she replied that she had spent a few hours on it already. Not true.

I made sure to pack and send fifty of her favorite CDs and the compact Bose radio/player. Nope. She had a small TV and cable connection. The remote caused a problem for a bit (I still have trouble navigating the remotes in my own household), so I ordered the senior-friendly Flipper Big Button remote. It was supposed to make things simpler, but instead she began unplugging every wire from every connection anytime she wanted something turned off. She could not figure out how to plug anything back in, so she went without until a family member visited and discovered the disconnect.

Mom was never a big reader though she went through a two-year obsession with the *New Yorker*. She always preferred periodicals to books. Then, no reading at all. Many who suffer from dementia have trouble with reading and comprehension as the disease progresses, so they are forced to give it up.

What is left to *do*?

Mom enjoys our time going to the mall, to lunch, to shop. But because her short-term memory is gone, she looks to me for companionship and entertainment immediately after we've spent four or five hours together. She is in a constant state of "what have you done for me lately?" and I am in a perpetual state of guilt because I can't do enough. Mom can't recall what we did or where we went or that an outing even took place. She lives in the moment, nothing more, nothing less ... until she obsesses over where she is going to live, when she can get her car back, when she can get her life back. "What did I do wrong?" she asks.

Quite by accident, she has found her purpose among her peers. She is attentive and comforting to everyone on the floor. She senses their grief or frustration and is immediately drawn to comfort them. Her presence has become her purpose. She has always liked being in control. Perhaps becoming the resident caregiver for the floor allows her to see herself in a staff role versus, as she would say, a "demented old resident" role. Mom makes sure to remind us that she is more hip, stylish, and spry than most of the old people around her.

But how to fill the hours?

In *The Philosophy of Loyalty*, the late American philosopher Josiah Royce asks what we all need to feel our life is worthwhile. The answer, he believes, is a cause beyond ourselves. The cause could be large (family, country, principle) or small (a building, project, the care of a pet). The important thing is that we give our lives meaning when we ascribe value to the cause and see it as worth making sacrifices for. Royce calls this dedication to a cause "loyalty" and regards it as the opposite of individualism.

Several organizations are emerging with creative ways to engage and delight those with dementia and their caregivers.

RESOURCES TO ENHANCE THE PRESENT

Alive Inside
www.aliveinside.org:
>A program featuring young people giving elders the gift of music.

Arts and Minds
artsandminds.org:
>A nonprofit committed to improving quality of life for people with dementia through art-centered programs.

Being in the Moment
beinginthemoment.org:
>Free tips, knowledge, suggestions, ideas, and coping mechanisms to help families and friends of people with dementia get through a day.

DAWN Method
thedawnmethod.com:
>A kind, strength-based, person-centered approach to dementia care that trains families and caregivers to maximize skills that dementia patients retain.

Dementia Action Alliance
daanow.org:
>A nonprofit devoted to providing hope and information about living proactively with dementia.

Opening Minds through Art (OMA)
scrippsoma.org:
>A group that fosters friendships between people with dementia and volunteers through art-making.

Silver Sneakers
tools.silversneakers.com:
>Live online fitness programs offered through Medicare Advantage plans.

TimeSlips

www.timeslips.org:
> Approaches that help elders with dementia shift away from the expectations of memory into a world of imagination.

When I was pregnant with my first child, I relied heavily on my copy of *What to Expect When You're Expecting* to guide me through the experience. Someone recently commented that we don't have a *What to Expect With Aging Parents* book. Hopefully this book will help. After having several kids and surviving the sleepless toddler years, I saw the same patterns emerge as I began caring for my mother: Did she need a snack or a nap? What was her mood like? Could we get her to shower or put on clean clothes?

I turned to the resources I used a decade earlier to find activities I could attend with my mother. I wanted to take her out and about and do things, but adult conversation and attention span were not what they used to be. The bonus factor that she loves babies and toddlers meant Hulafrog and Macaroni KID[95] became go-to websites. I found both franchises thorough and fun.

---

95 hulafrog.com/about-us

NOTED DEMENTIA CARE SPECIALISTS

Spending the highest quality time with Mom meant learning what leaders and thinkers in the dementia field are offering and saying. These pros include speech language pathologists, who assess brain function in rehab after a fall or an incident. The therapy they offer encompasses so much more than swallowing. Speech is a very complicated task that requires quite a bit of brain coordination. I found these resources helpful:

Adria Thompson
www.belightcare.com:
Dementia consultant and speech language pathologist.

Jessie Hillock
www.thememorycompass.com:
Dementia navigation coach, certified dementia practitioner, and speech language pathologist.

Tam Cummings, PhD
tamcummings.com:
Gerontologist and author of four books about dementia, including *Untangling Alzheimer's: The Guide for Families and Professionals*. She also offers training, consulting, and speaking, all to advance her goal of inspiring, educating, and empowering dementia caregivers.

Teepa Snow
teepasnow.com:
An extremely well-known and well-liked dementia care specialist. Her Positive Approach to Care (PAC) Team trains many caregivers in how to interact with those who suffer from dementia in a positive, understanding way. She is known for saying, "Dementia doesn't rob someone of their dignity; it is our reaction to them that does."

CARE FOR THE CAREGIVER / SELF-CARE AND RESPITE CARE

Caregiving can feel thankless, relentless, confusing, and exhausting. Just as you get into a groove, the symptoms change, a beloved staff member leaves, or an aide moves away. What curveball or crisis will pop up next? I feel like I am still living a reality version of whack-a-mole.

But I am extremely selfish about self-care. I also have Nancy as a trusted companion, confidant, and sounding board on this journey. We utilize our strengths to work together to provide comfort and care for Mom. No matter how much of your time, your energy, and your love you devote to caregiving, you have to reserve some love and care for yourself. If you don't make time for it, you can be certain nobody else will. And who is going to pick up the slack when you get sick and run-down?

In fall 2022 Nancy left to spend two weeks in Europe—a well-deserved break. That morning Mom called her multiple times. Despite her flights and layovers, Nancy talked to Mom briefly to settle her down. Then I got four voice mails in a row.

1:16 p.m.
Hi Nicole, call me when you can. Something's gotta change here or I'm gone. I don't know what else to say. I can't do this shit anymore. Thanks. Bye.

1:23 p.m.
I *need* to see somebody *here*, in my bedroom, whatever the hell room you have. Please give me a call.

1:40 p.m.
Hey Nicole, call me when you have time please. I'm trying to sort a couple things out. Thank you.

1:49 p.m.
Hi, it's Mom. I'm still trying to reach you. When you get time, give me a call and don't listen to Nancy cuz she doesn't know what she's talking about. I mean I don't know what she talks about with me anyway but I am having a really hard time. I need to go somewhere. I think I know what to do. I just want to talk it through with somebody and then get the hell out of here. I would really appreciate hearing from ya'. Let me know, thanks, love you.

I was running errands when I finally saw the messages. I called Mom back and reviewed "the plan" with her again: she would move to Arizona with us once we found a house and it would take time but we would get there. She calmed down. I told her to write "the plan" on a paper where she would see it frequently, if she could.

At that time she had been obsessed about the house and the car again. Nancy and I both told her that she'd lost her license because of the diagnosis and that her granddaughter had the car, so it stayed in the family. Mom seemed to be comforted with some answers and didn't get too angry about her losses.

That very day, however, she called me again:

6:08 p.m.
Nicole, hi, it's Mom. I just wanted to make sure we were on the same page in terms of talking about the sale of *my* house and things like that because I'm the one that has to make those decisions and I am pretty sure of what I'm going to do in all aspects of it so ... then I heard that *Sarah* had my car, which is not bad but somebody should've talked to me about it. I don't quite like the way some things are going, so I wanted to talk to you and let you know that and I wanted you to be on the watch for it. So call me and tell me who else I need to get in touch with because I'm gonna be moving and I'm gonna move to the East Coast so, you know, I don't need any more [sigh]. Anyway, just call me. Thanks. Bye.

Mom seemed to be hyperfocused on the sale of her house and car. She didn't remember that her license was revoked and rarely recalled that she currently lived on the East Coast in Maryland. We had been blessed with springtime, summer, and fall, but we were bracing for the coming winter because Mom does not like the cold. We weren't sure why Mom had become defiant and demanding again. But we saw that whenever we went over the logistics of where she lived and "the plan," she calmed down and was very gracious and appreciative, temporarily anyway.

I appeased her again by telling her she would move to Arizona with us the very next summer. No one could know what her mental state and health would be at that time, so we figured we would reassess accordingly. Thankfully, though, Mom was secure and safe in memory care even if she complained, as she often did, that she wasn't where she was supposed to be or wanted to be.

I know she is in the best possible place for her and for us. I see friends struggling with parents who want to stay in their home. Try as they might, my friends cannot find reliable aides or the consistent services their parents need. Since the pandemic many people have shifted careers, leaving a dire shortage of workers in every field. Aging in place is a very healthy and appealing choice, but as with all choices, it has pros and cons.

I spoke to Mom more often when Nancy was away, which was understandable. Nancy was always her first dial. I was a close second. Even so, Mom never wanted to stay on the phone more than five minutes, just long enough to be reassured about "the plan" and express her gratitude. After we hung up, she forgot everything again.

One of the Mayo Clinic books I read, *Mayo Clinic on Alzheimer's Disease and Other Dementias*, cited the concept of emotional memory.[96] People with dementia may not have much short-term memory, but they remember how you make them feel. You know the quote from Maya Angelou: "I've learned that people will forget what you said, people will forget what you did, but people will never forget how you made them feel."

We noticed a significant increase in Mom's frustration and calls when Nancy was away in Europe. I drove down for a quick visit but she noticeably missed the frequency of Nancy's presence in her routine.

The very nature of dementia is trying for both your parent and you. There's a name for what you're feeling: caregiver syndrome, defined as the impact that caring for an ill or dying loved one has on your physical, mental, and emotional well-being. According to Parenting Our Parents, which helps families with aging seniors navigate the system, caregiver syndrome is a term that acknowledges your "relentless fatigue, shock of diagnosis, change in roles from partner to nurse, guilt, resentment, depression, and outright grieving as you watch your loved one failing and in pain."[97]

Most who ride the roller coaster of caregiving stress and fatigue are women since, as the Institute on Aging has calculated, upwards of 75 percent of all caregivers are female.[98]

The good news is that help is abundant. Google "help for caregivers of the elderly" and you'll get literally millions of hits connecting you to everything from programs and advice to

---

96 www.amazon.com/Clinic-Alzheimers-Disease-Other-Dementias/dp/1893005615
97 parentingourparents.org/70-of-all-caregivers-over-the-age-of-70-die-first-recognizing-and-responding-to-caregiver-syndrome/
98 www.caregiver.org/resource/caregiver-statistics-demographics/

resources and support services. Use them because caregiving can compromise your health. Caregivers take more prescription medications, including those for anxiety and depression, than others in their age group.[99]

And don't forget "respite care," relief for primary caregivers that can be as short as an afternoon or as long as several weeks. This care for caregivers can be provided at home or an adult care center. Some assisted living facilities that cater to the elderly also have space, or even a wing, where caregivers can rest and recharge. In some instances respite care can do double duty: it can help the caregiver and give them a chance to sample life at the facility.

Our Story: Thirty Minutes of Exercise

Exercise has always been my primary means of stress relief. I have made it a standard daily habit since I was a teenager. I did step aerobics and yoga up until the very day of delivery with every one of my kids. I prioritize thirty minutes of vigorous exercise every day. I jog if the weather is nice, pop in an exercise DVD, or flow through a yoga routine. I pack my running shoes and workout gear every time I travel. Exercise has been proven to improve mood. It also prompts me to eat healthier, sleep better, and flush out toxins and stress. Walking is one of the best exercise methods around. If you are stuck indoors due to caregiving, you can march in place.

---

[99] www.webmd.com/depression/stress-and-depression/

RESOURCES FOR CAREGIVERS

ARCH National Respite Network and Resource Center
archrespite.org:
>Organization that helps develop respite and crisis care programs.

Caregiver Action Network
www.caregiveraction.org:
>A national family caregiver organization whose mission is improving quality of life for the more than ninety million Americans who care for loved ones with chronic conditions, disabilities, disease, or the frailties of old age.

MOVIES FOR CAREGIVERS

Here Today, a hilarious and touching 2021 film with Billy Crystal and Tiffany Haddish about friendship, family, and humor in dealing with a dementia diagnosis.

I Care a Lot, a 2020 thriller/comedy and cautionary tale featuring Rosamund Pike, Dianne Wiest, and Peter Dinklage about a clever court-appointed guardian who uses the system to swindle elders out of their assets.

Robin's Wish, a 2020 American documentary film that offers a look into the life and final days of Robin Williams and how his struggles with Lewy body dementia impacted his acting career and contributed to him taking his life.

Ruth, a 2021 twelve-minute dark and dramatic film that follows an elderly woman with dementia who becomes lost in her memories and her deteriorating home.

Ruth, a 2023 nine-minute short film about a working woman caring for her elderly mother at home.

Still Alice, a 2014 drama film based on the 2007 novel by neuroscientist Lisa Genova, which features fifty-year-old Alice Howland, a cognitive psychology professor at Harvard University and a world-renowned linguistics expert who suffers early-onset Alzheimer's disease.

Stutz, a 2022 Netflix documentary that pays tribute to Paul Stutz, the psychiatrist of filmmaker Jonah Hill who reveals in an interview that he has Parkinson's disease.[100]

The Savages, a 2007 drama/comedy featuring Philip Seymour Hoffman and Laura Linney as siblings who get a crisis call and struggle to deal with their dad, even without having spouses or children in the mix to complicate the situation.

Wine, Women, & Dementia, a 2023 documentary that reveals the isolation, financial stress, and physical and emotional toll dementia takes on family caregivers and their afflicted loved ones. The trailer reads, "It's a roadtrip connecting

---

100 www.nytimes.com/2022/11/15/movies/stutz-review.html

the disconnected because until there's a cure, there's community."[101]

You're Not You, a 2014 drama chronicling the struggle of a classical pianist diagnosed with ALS, played by Hilary Swank, and the brash college student who becomes her caregiver.

SUPPORT FOR CAREGIVERS

AARP
www.aarp.org:
An American interest and advocacy group that addresses issues affecting people over the age of fifty.

AgingCare
www.agingcare.com:
A directory that connects families with in-home care and senior housing.

Alzwell Caregiver Support
www.alzwell.com:
An online magazine that serves as a heartfelt, practical resource for Alzheimer's disease and dementia caregivers.

Anti-Aging Games
www.anti-aginggames.com:
A website that offers games designed to improve memory and focusing skills.

Assured Allies
www.assuredallies.com:
A company that assesses how a person is aging, develops a personalized Successful Aging Plan and a set of targeted interventions, and provides an aging coach to help see the plan through. Free to individuals through long-term care insurance companies.

---
101 www.winewomenanddementia.com

DailyCaring
dailycaring.com:
> A caregiving website that offers practical solutions for the day-to-day challenges of those who care for someone fifty or older and the 14.9 million people who care for someone living with Alzheimer's disease or dementia.

Daughterhood
www.daughterhood.org:
> A community of people who support each other in caring for aging parents. Daughterhood offers virtual support Circles focused on connection or specific topics to support and build confidence in people providing care.

Family Caregiver Alliance
www.caregiver.org:
> An online support group for adults caring for their parents or other relatives that also provides a list of in-person support groups in different states.

Hilarity for Charity
www.wearehfc.org:
> A national nonprofit that cares for families impacted by Alzheimer's disease, inspires a new generation of advocates for Alzheimer's, and leads in brain health research and education.

Leeza's Care Connection
leezascareconnection.org:
> An organization founded by talk show host Leeza Gibbons, who also appeared on *Dancing with the Stars*. Leeza's mother had Alzheimer's and Leeza wanted to create what she "wished we had when we were going through this journey."

Love for Our Elders
loveforourelders.org/our-story:
> A team of more than fifty thousand volunteers across seventy countries who fight loneliness with love through letter writing, in-person volunteering events, and more.

My Pivotal Point
mypivotalpoint.com/caregiving-consulting:
> A consulting business that helps caregivers achieve a healthy balance among the three dimensions of their lives: personal, professional, and self.

Naborforce
naborforce.com/our-services:
> A platform to find vetted people in your community to help do things family and neighbors would do if they were available.

National Adult Day Services Association
www.nadsa.org/for-caregivers/choosing-a-center:
> An organization dedicated to advancing the development, recognition, and use of adult day services.

National Caregiving Foundation
caregivingfoundation.org:
> An organization that uses direct mail to inform the caregiving community about Alzheimer's disease, including warning signs and symptoms, and offers suggestions to caregivers, including those who care for wounded soldiers.

National Council on Aging
www.ncoa.org:
> A charitable organization that promotes healthy, equitable, financially secure aging nationwide.

Next Avenue
www.nextavenue.org:
> Public media's first and only national publication for older adults.

Rosalynn Carter Institute for Caregivers
rosalynncarter.org:
> An institute that champions family caregivers by building cross-sector partnerships, leading research projects and initiatives, developing and implementing programs, and advocating for public policy.

Today's Caregiver
caregiver.com:
> The first national magazine dedicated to caregivers, founded in 1995.

Top Ten Tips to Keep Your Brain Young
www.youtube.com/watch?v=2tcEgqTWbxQ:
> A TED Talk by Elizabeth Amini, CEO of Anti-Aging Games, referenced above.

Well Spouse Association
wellspouse.org:
> A nonprofit membership organization that addresses the needs of people caring for a chronically ill and/or disabled spouse or partner.

BOOKS FOR CAREGIVERS

AlzAuthors
alzauthors.com:
> A place to share Alzheimer's disease and dementia books, blogs, and stories and, in so doing, lift the silence and stigma of Alzheimer's and other dementias.

A Year of Self Care Journal: 52 Weeks to Cultivate Positivity & Joy
by Allison Task, MS, PCC (Rockridge Press, 2021)

PODCASTS FOR CAREGIVERS

Better Health While Aging: The Helping Older Parents Podcast
betterhealthwhileaging.net/series/hop

Daughterhood The Podcast: For Caregivers
thewholecarenetwork.com/daughterhood-the-podcast-for-caregivers

This Is Getting Old: Moving Towards an Age-Friendly World
melissabphd.com/podcast-blog/

Our Story: Unexpected Angels

January 2022

    When our parents became a couple, my stepsister Amy was eighteen years old and I was seven. Amy is the oldest of her siblings; I am the oldest of three. Our parents were married to other people when they met. Amy and I have very different perspectives on what happened and how the relationship between her father and my mother affected our respective families.

    Amy lived in LA for a short time after high school as the affair was beginning. She was living with cousins and working before going to college. I had just finished second grade. Our blended family adjusted over the years and I was closer to some stepsiblings than others. As I matured and became an adult, I grew closer to Amy.

    Amy met me in LA to help empty Mom's house to prepare it for sale. Mom had requested that she be present when we sorted through and donated items. My previous attempts to honor her request had proved disastrous. When she was in the psychiatric facility, we had a couple of weeks to get the house ready. We hoped the meds would stabilize her depression and agitation and allow her to transition into a senior living residence.

    Amy and I interrupted our packing and put Mom on speakerphone every time she called. Though the staff had taken her cell phone, the nurses had phone numbers for Nancy and me and allowed her to call us occasionally. She called from the community phone in the hallway. Sometimes a nurse would bring Mom a chair, other times she would sit on the floor. We sent her a bunch of warm clothes, socks, and puzzles. Family members were sending her cards.

It was difficult to hear her sound so defeated and miserable, suffering in an unfamiliar place among strangers in a cold climate she hated. The wrath of her domineering paranoia over the past six months was still raw and painful for me. I sympathized with her predicament. We had tried to work with her until we realized nothing would happen unless we took drastic measures.

Many of my friends were also dealing with aging parents. One friend shared her experience in helping her mother sort through belongings in an attempt to downsize. It was an exercise in one step forward, two steps back. It is difficult for any of us to let go of things that bring back a flood of memories. I hadn't been able to put a dent in clearing the clutter with Mom around, but I was able to make a mental inventory and formulate a rough plan that I put into action once she was on the opposite coast.

Amy and I had an incredible week of casual coworking to clear out the house. She sorted through the overwhelming number of papers and folders in the drawers, cupboards, and file cabinets. We are a family that enjoys sending greeting cards for all occasions, and Mom apparently had saved them all. We took breaks to visit the post office, walk to the store, and drop donations at charity organizations.

Mom had been the executor of my grandparents' estate. All the photos and keepsakes from her parents and their six children were there for review. So many pictures. Grandma had a Kodak Brownie box camera and used it often. The small square black-and-white photos with the scalloped edges are perfectly precious. Formal photos were taken in a studio and touched up with coloring.

I saved all the photos and mailed some to various cousins who I knew would appreciate them. We discovered photos of family reunions, class reunions, weddings, and endless envelopes of candid drugstore prints. It would have been easy to spend several days reading through letters and reminiscing, but we were rushed for time. Most of the random office documents went into the shred pile or the recycle bin.

I even came across my report cards from grammar school, my brother's adoption papers, foster parent papers, divorce papers, and a handwritten commencement speech given to the Notre Dame Class of 1875. I shipped several boxes of treasures to Nancy, whose memory is sharp and vivid. The document discovery sparked renewed interest in investigating and chronicling a family tree.

Amy left after one week due to other commitments, leaving me to finish the job. I dropped her at the airport. A bit deflated, I was still determined to persevere. My phone rang and my dad's number flashed on the screen. I debated whether to answer but picked up. He was groggy and sounded off. He explained that he had been transported to the hospital by ambulance due to vertigo. They were running tests to determine what kind. I immediately started bawling. Now both parents were in crisis. His condition turned out to be treatable and he was better in a few days. He later told me he had no recollection of calling me that morning. I wondered if he, too, had dementia.

Fortunately, his confusion was only temporary due to the medication they had given him.

I spent another week packing and sorting. The house had four bedrooms and the detached garage had six giant cabinets full of random things. I donated the holiday decorations, frames, pots, lawn chairs, boxes of tchotchkes, and doorknobs, yes doorknobs! I was thrilled to discover Grandma's candy dish, which I fondly remember filled with orange jelly slices, chocolate-covered peanuts, and what I called "pink Pepto Bismol candy pieces"—thick pink wintergreen Canada Mints. I bubble wrapped it and brought it home in my carry-on luggage to make sure it wasn't lost, broken, or forgotten.

An angel appeared in the form of a neighbor from across the street who taught me how to properly pack a kitchen and helped drive donation loads. I was grateful for her enthusiastic generosity and perfectly pleasant company. She made the week fly by and boosted my morale. Mom had always raved about the amazing camaraderie among the neighbors. I was thrilled to finally meet several in person after hearing about them for so many years. I also was thankful for the impromptu support. When such help shows up, accept it!

We got the job done and it was time to hand over the keys to another neighbor, a Realtor, to prep the house for sale. She organized the painters, landscapers, inspectors, handyman, stager, and photographer in preparation for putting the house on the market in the coming months. COVID-19 isolation didn't help Mom's mental state but we hoped we could benefit from the boost it bestowed on the real estate market. And wow, did we ever. The house ended up selling for significantly over asking, just before interest rates began to climb. We needed the cash to cover the horrendously expensive cost of memory care.

APPROACHING THE END

Our Story: Suicidal Threats

Mom grew up in the Midwest, surrounded by a cohesive community of family, friends, and neighbors. She was the fourth girl, followed by two younger brothers to make an even half dozen. The eldest was the brainiac, followed by the beauty, then Nurse Nancy, the tomboy athlete. Mom was very close to her brother, just eighteen months younger. The youngest child arrived a decade behind the rest of the brood. The Catholic Church was their touchstone. Their parents were active in the parish, and the children attended the Catholic K-12 school.

For most of her life, Mom had practiced her faith though she abandoned it when her father passed in 1995. The Catholic church forbids suicide and formerly would not allow funerals for those who had taken their own life.

Mom said she had considered slitting her wrists but didn't want to make a mess. She had also considered swallowing pills but didn't know which ones or how many to consume. She had proposed driving her car off a cliff but didn't want to hurt anyone else and she loved her car. She was unsure and afraid and didn't want to experience pain. She and her brother nearly drowned in a river when she was a young child. She reflected on how peaceful she felt as she floated and felt her consciousness slipping, but she forever feared the water after that incident. She also declared that she could simply stop eating and slowly waste away. A few hours later she inevitably got hungry and ate a snack.

Mom was never fond of old people and didn't like their decrepit posture, constant chatter about aches and ailments, wrinkled skin, and polyester clothes. She never wanted to grow old. She knows she has arrived but places herself in another category—aged but not old. She explained to me that she had lived a good life and that when her mind began to change, she had started plotting her ultimate demise.

I certainly didn't want to lose Mom, but I pondered what I might do if I developed dementia. Would I realize it and have the courage to take action before I lost the capacity to take matters into my own hands? That scenario plays out in the film *Still Alice*. Evidence is still very murky on how much heredity, lifestyle, or anything plays a part in who will experience the slow burn in the brain. Knowing Mom and her personality and her previous and current statements about being over and done with life made me see her side clearly.

Mom said over and over that she was ready to go. Some family members struggled with the mention of suicide. Many people are very wary of discussing the subject. Nancy, still very steeped in her faith, believes we all have a purpose whether we are aware of it or not. Nancy and I both believe Mom's presence is her purpose.

This zany journey of doctor visits, phone calls, flights, arguments, exasperation, and exhaustion had finally landed us in a place of peace. Mom is not entirely happy where she landed and still reminds us of this fact daily. Nancy and I are relieved, however, and we became closer as we both recovered and became care companions for Mom.

COMFORT CARE: PALLIATIVE CARE VERSUS HOSPICE

Palliative care can be equated to comfort care. Its focus is helping people manage pain and discomfort as they endure a chronic illness or terminal condition. Palliative care enlists caregivers trained in massage, meditation, counseling, nutrition, and spiritual support for all faiths. It can be administered in the hospital or at home. A patient can pursue aggressive treatment and receive palliative care simultaneously.

Typically, medical professionals want to save or heal or cure a patient through prescriptions, tests, procedures, and surgery. Sometimes families realize their loved one may not return to the level of cognition they had before the stroke, the fall, or the surgery. A new baseline is established. They want to maintain their loved one's dignity, manage discomfort, and prevent complications, so they request palliative care.

Hospice care is a form of palliative care offered to patients who have decided they no longer wish to pursue potential curative treatment and prefer a calm, organic environment as they near the end of life. A patient is admitted to hospice when their physician determines they have less than six months to live. Hospice in general is usually covered by Medicare, but not entirely.[102]

Patients on hospice are treated through methods that provide comfort, mitigate pain, and alleviate nausea. They may continue taking medication for certain conditions, such as heart disease, but cease medication for their terminal condition, which sometimes changes the biological dynamic. Patients have the option to come off hospice care if their health improves.

Palliative care has been shown to make patients happier with the care they receive and to cost less because it reduces the need for hospitalizations and emergency room trips.[103]

Sometimes the patient is ready to let it all go, but their mother, spouse, or friend may persuade them to keep fighting. Some people don't want a hospice team to emotionally prepare them for their loved one's imminent passing. Instead they never give up hope that one more critical trial or off-label treatment will produce a miracle.

Barbara Bush and Jimmy Carter are two prominent figures who chose hospice over further treatment. One could argue they lived long and quite productive lives. Every life is different, every disease is different, each decision is different. But everyone

---
102 www.medicare.gov/coverage/hospice-care
103 stateline.org/2017/07/10/why-some-patients-arent-getting-palliative-care/

is helped when they know the options and have the tough discussions beforehand.

Dementia is one of the most common diseases and conditions associated with hospice care, according to the National Hospice and Palliative Care Organization. But when is it time for hospice? One healthcare system offers questions to ask:

1. **Is the patient or loved one showing signs of decline?** Are curative treatments no longer working? Has the patient decided to stop testing and hospitalizations? Is the patient able to perform activities of daily living? Have they lost 10 percent or more of their body weight, or had more than three hospitalizations, in the past four to six months?

2. **Have you taken the patient's wishes into consideration?** They should be easy to know if their preferences are spelled out in an advanced care plan, a living will, or a durable power of attorney for healthcare or, in some states, a Five Wishes document.[104]

Most patients don't enroll in hospice until their time of death is very near. Half of patients who sign up pass away within three weeks while 35.7 percent die within a week.[105]

Our Story: A Stepfather's Last Days

I had a brief experience with hospice when my stepfather passed away. He had smoked for decades and developed lung cancer in his mid-sixties. He underwent chemo and radiation for several months, which helped but did not destroy the cancer. When it returned a short time later, it had metastasized to his brain. He chose to stop treatment and elected to enter hospice care at home.

The children, stepchildren, and some grandchildren gathered at my mother and stepfather's home in California. We all had

---

104 www.vitas.com/hospice-and-palliative-care-basics/when-is-it-time-for-hospice/is-it-time-for-hospice-3-questions-to-ask-yourself
105 home.liebertpub.com/publications/journal-of-palliative-medicine/41

meaningful individual final farewell conversations with him. He was not afraid. He was only sixty-seven, but he had lived a life full of family and friends and a career as a counselor and communicator who centered his practice around positive self-esteem. We all benefited from his attention and guidance.

During his final days, he remained in the hospital bed set up in the living room. We wandered in and out as we chased the kids and chatted with each other, prepared meals, and waited for the inevitable. One sunny afternoon his limbs began to turn blue and his breathing pattern changed. We were summoned to his bedside. About a dozen of us encircled his bed as he passed peacefully.

DEATH DOULAS

Death doulas, who are trained and certified by various organizations, are part of a growing number of support staff who assist the aging population. They offer social and emotional support for the family and the patient during this difficult time. They also can offer respite for an exhausted caregiver. Doula fees are typically a private pay expense that can cost anywhere from fifty to more than one hundred dollars per hour.

Some doulas are trained in massage therapy, mindfulness and/or meditation. They can also facilitate discussions on practical matters, including expressing wishes for peace and comfort near the end. Does the patient desire silence or soft music? Are there certain friends or family members they would like near and others from whom they'd rather steer clear? Different relationships bring different energy into the space and emotions and opinions run high during these times. A doula can help soothe egos and handle hurt by preserving what the patient wants when others forget amid their grief and goodbyes.

Life really does come full circle. Birth doulas help expecting mothers draft a birth plan as a guideline going into the birth. Circumstances can and do change, but the plan is there as a baseline and a preparation process. The same goes for an end-of-life plan. Discussing it may be difficult, but better to have peace than panic during the final days or weeks. Have the conversation. Ask, ask, ask, and respect your parent's wishes.

RESOURCES FOR END OF LIFE

Addio
www.ouraddio.com:
> Comprehensive, nimble end-of-life estate planning process that makes it easy to change documents.

Compassion and Choices
compassionandchoices.org/our-issues/dementia-end-of-life-care:
> A nonprofit that advocates for and tracks legislation in states where medical aid in dying is authorized in the US.

Death Café
deathcafe.com:
> A nonprofit that arranges death cafes, events at which people drink tea, eat cake, and discuss death, the goal being to help people make the most of their lives.

Dementia with Dignity
www.thedawnmethod.com:
> A network headed by Judy Cornish, a geriatric care manager and elder law attorney, that trains loved ones and professionals in care methods that provide a supportive experience for dementia patients at home.

Dignitas
www.dignitas.ch:
> An organization in Switzerland that offers physician-assisted suicide. Amy Bloom's book, *In Love. A Memoir of Love and Loss*, addresses this experience, which her husband chose when he was diagnosed with early-onset Alzheimer's.

Hospice Hustle
www.propublica.org/article/how-to-research-your-hospice-and-avoid-hospice-fraud:
> A ProPublica special report for readers, patients, and caregivers on how to avoid problems and fraud in the hospice industry.

International End-of-Life Doula Association
inelda.org:
>An organization that trains end-of-life doulas and provides a searchable compendium of certified doulas.

Our Story: A Life of Plateaus

As of this writing, Mom is safe and well cared for in a memory care residence. When I mention Mom has dementia, many people ask me, "Does she know who you are?" She most definitely does. Sometimes she confuses Nancy and me when she is leaving voice mails. She is still able to use her phone when she remembers to charge it and doesn't lose it. I could write another chapter on that subject alone.

Mom has experienced significant loss in her short-term memory. If I leave for three minutes to use the bathroom, she forgets I am there for a visit. She is still able to perform all of her Activities of Daily Living (ADLs), with some encouragement from the staff on showering. I would currently put Mom in the moderate to advanced Alzheimer's category. One nurse described many eldercare ailments as a series of declines and plateaus, with a new baseline established each time, because these diseases are progressive. There is rarely a return to the original baseline of ability. Ceasing some or all medications, as directed by a doctor or hospice, can sometimes create a seemingly miraculous recovery or resurgence of cognitive ability. These are rare and usually fleeting.

Mom complains about where she lives and the people in the unit. She claims she does not belong where all the old people live. She does, however, experience a notable sense of comfort when we return to the facility after a brief outing. Even though she can't picture where she lives when we are out and about, she recognizes it when we cruise into the parking lot. Maybe that has to do with her emotional memory; she remembers how the place makes her feel.

We are in the midst of the promised move to Arizona. I will find another exceptional memory care environment near our new home. I don't know if another major move will cause her distress. It will be an adjustment for everyone. She will, however, be back in the sunshine and warmer weather, which I think she will appreciate.

She will also be closer to more family members in Arizona, which will be beneficial for all of us. We have no idea how or when the brain erosion will progress to the point of hindering more of her physical capabilities. We are grateful for the resources we have and the power of the baby boomer generation that, by its sheer size, will change the landscape of care in the coming years.

Mom still never waivers on her commitment to making the world better for women. I had her vintage "ERA NOW" T-shirt made into a pillow for her birthday. The penchant for advocacy that she instilled in me is helping her now. It is what drives my work on her behalf. It is what drives her to help those around her, wherever she is. Hopefully, it will help her continue to live a fulfilling life despite having dementia. We will continue to adjust our expectations as her condition plateaus and declines.

CIRCLE OF LIFE

You know the physical, emotional, and financial toll that caring for your parent is having on you. If you do not already have a plan in place for yourself and your family, maybe your experiences as a caregiver will motivate you to do so. Heed the quote from wellness educator Joyce Sunada, "If you don't take time for your wellness, you will be forced to take time for your illness."[106] Life is unfair, life is uncertain. Planning and prevention are the pathways to a better future for yourself and your loved ones. Don't wait and hire professionals when necessary.

You can start by setting up a wise insurance landscape for yourself.

It would be nice if *Sesame Street* could have Grover or Cookie Monster explain the alphabet according to Medicare. Most of us end up feeling like Oscar the Grouch when dealing with the Medicare bureaucracy. Though the program is federal, plans are also state specific. There are many Medicare advisors available to help; some are licensed to work in multiple states.

The alphabet soup of coverage options begins with Medicare Part A (hospital insurance) and Medicare Part B (medical insurance), the basics. Medicare Part D is more readily memorable: think of "D" for drug coverage.

Medicare Part C (supplemental insurance) comprises bundled Medicare Advantage plans that combine benefits for hospital care, medical treatment, doctor visits, and prescription drugs.

---

[106] www.union-bulletin.com/local_columnists/sound_mind_sound_body/make-time-for-wellness-to-avoid-making-time-for-illness/article_1cb7bf64-c7a3-11eb-8d13-e30f3afd0dee.html

Some include add-on coverage for dental, vision, and hearing. There are pros and cons to Medicare Advantage plans as well as associated costs.

Medigap is an alternative to Advantage plans.[107] It is another insurance layer, offered through private insurance companies and designed to fill in the gaps where Medicare falls short. You pay premiums for this secondary insurance to help pay for copays and deductibles. There are many different options and some are only available in certain areas. Since every situation is individual, discuss your situation with your local agent.

No one knows better than you the firsthand care experiences that come with living at home versus living at an assisted living residence. So why not give yourself some options when your time comes? Consider rounding out your own healthcare coverage with a fifth part. Call it Medicare Part U (you), a long-term care plan.[108]

RESOURCES FOR CHOOSING INSURANCES

Medicare
www.medicare.gov

National Association of Benefits and Insurance Professionals (NABIP)
nabip.org/looking-for-an-agent/find-an-agent

State Health Insurance Assistance Programs
shiphelp.org

US Centers for Medicare & Medicaid Services
cms.gov

---

107 www.medicare.gov/health-drug-plans/medigap
108 www.aarp.org/membership/benefits/healthcare/long-term-care/

YOU ARE NOT ALONE

Millions upon millions of people around the world are going through some version of what you are experiencing right now. Each situation has unique players and challenges, but as Bob, the lawyer, so wisely put it, "Same play, different actors."

The good news is that the incidence of dementia is already too big to be ignored. Some people are scrambling, some are innovating, others are collaborating to find ways to surf this tsunami, or at least stay afloat without getting sucked under.

The resources you need are out there, but it takes effort to find the ones that are right for you. We know caregiving is all consuming and leaves little energy for extra effort to do anything else. So ask for help. I am a doer. Find a doer near you and don't be afraid to ask. I was in sales for part of my career so I know the worst that can happen: they can say no.

On the other hand, the worst that can happen if you don't ask for help is that you will erode your own well-being and health and perhaps even die. Look at the statistics for caregiver mortality. Is that the statistic you want to be?

Hopefully, this book has given you at least one starting point to research resources that might be right for your situation. You are a caregiver. Don't forget to take care of yourself, too.

ACKNOWLEDGMENTS

I could not have survived these last few years with my sanity intact without the love, laughter, and guidance of my Aunt Nancy, aka Nurse Nancy, a brilliant and nurturing caregiver and companion throughout this dementia ordeal. Our relationship flourished through this experience and I am grateful.

I am thankful for my bean counter husband whose expertise in tax, accounting, and investment affairs helped us navigate the financial aspects of selling Mom's house and covering her care costs. He also graciously supports my push to self-publish our story to help others.

I am thankful for my dad and his easy wit and humor as well as his patience when I nudge him into getting his important documents in order.

We can take professional pride in publishing this book because of my editor, Lorraine Ash, a genius with decades of experience who I consider a close personal friend. I must also thank Diane Lang for introducing me to Lorraine. Never underestimate the power of your personal and professional network. I am a networking fiend. The best connections come through casual conversation in a synergistic, serendipitous fashion.

My incredibly creative niece, Kristen Graham Brown, founder and owner of Hoot Design Company, designed the book cover that perfectly captures the confusion many families face in dealing with dementia and eldercare. Many thanks to my stepsisters, too, for continuing to ask after and care for my mom.

I thank Christopher Kellogg of Nightingale NJ for enhancing my eldercare education with his kind, calm demeanor and extensive experience in the senior space. I am also grateful for the entire Daughterhood team and community for sharing their stories and for their continuing efforts to bring attention to, and inspire advocacy for, caregivers everywhere.

Many thanks to my friends who support me in whatever I choose to do and pursue. And to my children, who keep me humble by questioning every piece of advice I offer. I am blessed beyond words.

Printed in the USA
CPSIA information can be obtained
at www.ICGtesting.com
JSHW061151151124
73596JS00006B/14